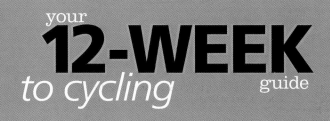

your 12-WEEK to cycling guide

FROM YOUR ARMCHAIR TO A 25 KM RACE IN 12 WEEKS

by Daniel Ford

Training programme by Adam Dickson

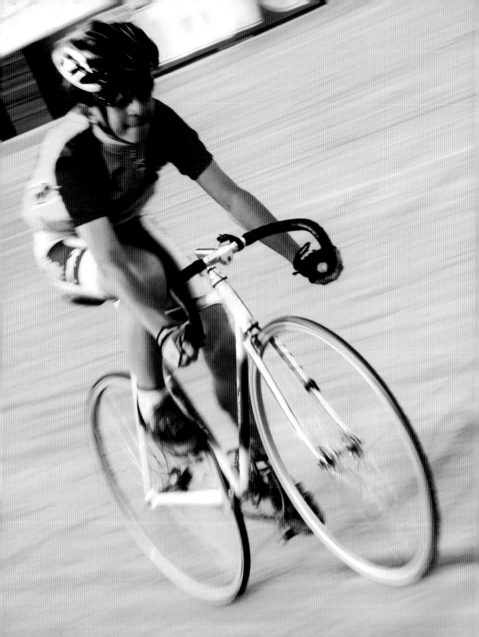

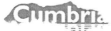
your 12-WEEK to cycling guide

FROM YOUR ARMCHAIR TO A 25 KM RACE IN 12 WEEKS

Fact box sources (note: conversions are from g to oz (US) and from ml to fl oz (US). (1) UK Department of Health. (2) USGS. (3) UK Department of Health. (4) UK Department of Health: Sport and Exercise Medicine: a Fresh Approach (2012). (5) McDonald's, Pizza Hut, KFC (all US). (6) P Lally, European Journal of Social Psychology. (7) US National Health Interview Survey (2010). (8) Harvard Heart Letter (July 2004). (9) Coca-Cola (US), Starbucks (US). (10) UK Department of Health: Start Active, Stay Active (2011) and US The President's Council on Physical Fitness and Sport. (11) UK Department of Health: Start Active, Stay Active (2011) and www.bootsdiets.com. (12) US National Sleep Foundation. (13) UK NHS Sport and Exercise Medicine: A Fresh Approach (2011). (14) US The President's Council on Physical Fitness and Sports: Fast Facts About Sports Nutrition. (15) Drinkaware.co.uk. (16) US The President's Council on Physical Fitness and Sports: Fast Facts About Sports Nutrition. (17) US The President's Council on Physical Fitness and Sports: Exercise and Weight Control. (18) AM Williamson and AM Feyer, British Medical Journal (2000). (19) USGS. (20) Fitness Australia. (21) *Triathlon: Serious About Your Sport* (NHP). (22) Olaf Lahl et al, University of Dusseldorf (2008). (23) JH Stubbe et al, The association between exercise participation and well-being (2006) and various others. Photos: iStockphoto.com and www.sxc.hu, P19 Guenter M Kirchweger, www.redfloor.at. P20 Luke Todd, www.salladhor.devaiantart.com. P29 Scott Moore, www.typer.ca~sqm. P30 Luke Todd, www.salladhor.devaiantart.com. P36 Torli Roberts. P39 Thad Zajdowicz. P40 Leswek Nowak. P46 Hans Thoursie, www.serpentino.se. P49 Philip MacKenzie, www.photoshowcase.co.uk. P57 Päivi Rytivaara. P58 Sebastian Kapciak, http://home.elka.pw.edu.pl/~skapciak/. P62 Mateusz Kapciak, introgic. P64 Thad Zajdowicz. P67 roxinasz. P68 Scott Moore, www.typer.ca~sqm. P72 Christa Richert, RGBStock.com, www.rgbstock.com/user/ayla87. P77 Samantha Villagran, www.winkgallery.com. P78 Gabriela Ruellan. P84 Dominik Gwarek, www.kikashi.webpages. pl. P87 Catalin Stratila. P88 Nico van Diem. P104 Nuno Fernandes, http://photodetail.blogspot. com. P106 Svetlana Maksimovic. P109 Bill Owen, www.eyestir.com. P110 Luke Todd, www.salladhor. devaiantart.com. P113 Leswek Nowak. P119 Wojtek Mysliwiec, www.hightechstudios.com. P123 Luke Todd, www.salladhor.devaiantart.com. P140 Pawel Zawistowski, www.milionporad.pl. P143 Marcos Santos.

your 12-WEEK plan

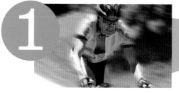

1

Commit to the challenge

You need to tell others about your plans…

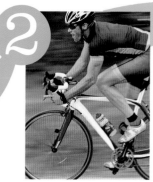

2

Hit the road

So far, so good. Now, after the mental preparation, it's time to get moving…

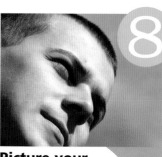

8

Picture your success

Look ahead to your 25 km ride and see yourself completing it in style…

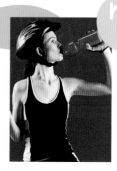

7

You're well on your way

Think back and congratulate yourself on how far you have come already…

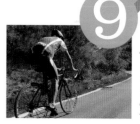

9

The end is in sight

It's time to push on towards the finish…

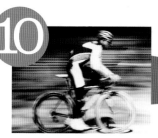

10

Focus on your goal

Beware the spectre of over-confidence. It can kill all your hard work…

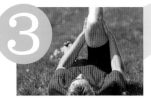

3
Rest well and stretch
Get good sleep, stretch often, and treat rest days with respect…

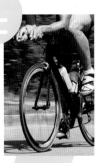

4
Make cycling a habit
Before you know it cycling will be part of your life…

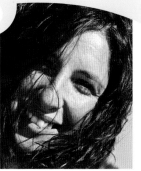

6
Fitness benefits
Trust your subconscious. It will work to give you plenty of benefits from your training…

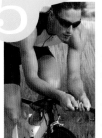

5
Enjoy smooth cycling
Concentrate on a smooth pedal stroke to fully enjoy cycling…

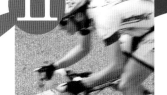

11
Now ease up
With your challenge day so close you can start winding down…

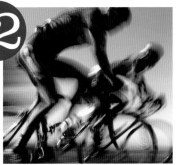

12
Get ready to ride
After many weeks of hard training you are ready…

introduction

Your challenge starts here...

We can tell from your fine choice of reading material that you are a person who knows what you want. The mere fact you have this book in your hands and are reading it, means you have probably already made the most important step: deciding to get out of your armchair and train for a 25 km (15.5 miles) cycle ride.

How many times have you heard that the, "First step is the most important," or the only way to complete a project is to, "Stop delaying and get started". Well, you can comfort yourself that by making the decision to follow the programme means you are already on your way!

A cycle ride of 25 km can seem a long way if you haven't been out riding for a long time (have you dusted off your bicycle yet?). But while it's important you always keep your eyes on the end goal, treat the programme as a series of smaller challenges. First you make the decision to do it (check), then you get exercising (a few gentle rides), then you start ticking off the weeks one by one. It's a lot easier to tackle a smaller task, then another, en route to a big task, than it is to try to mentally bite off the whole thing in

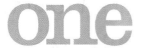

There is only one thing you should be concentrating on right now and that is to start exercising. Don't attempt to give up smoking and drinking, and start eating salads just yet. You are more likely to give up if you try to change too much at once.

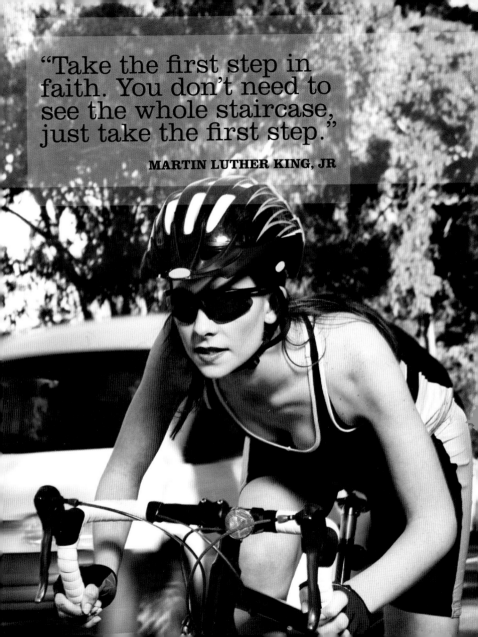

"Take the first step in faith. You don't need to see the whole staircase, just take the first step."

MARTIN LUTHER KING, JR

one go. So put any worries you may have to one side, get started, and keep chipping away.

Everyone will have their own motivator for taking on this cycle challenge. You may want to start training to lose a bit of weight or to tone up your leg muscles. You may simply have decided you have had enough of feeling sluggish during the day and need to get fit again. Or maybe the teasing from a friend that, "You could never do it," finally got too much.

Whatever you own personal reason is, always remember to keep focused on the cycle challenge and not on your motivator. If you keep worrying you are not losing weight as fast as you hoped, then you are likely to become dispirited and give up altogether. Rather, you should keep working on the small steps in the programme and congratulate yourself on the progress you are making with that. The other factors, such as weight loss, feeling energized during the day, and so on, will look after themselves naturally as you get fitter.

Another important step at this early stage is to visualize your success. It is good to imprint your future success into your mind, as this will help guide your body through the coming weeks.

You can do this more or less anywhere, but it does help your concentration if you find somewhere quiet

hear

Listen to your body. You know when you are feeling good and you know when you are not because your body tells you. Follow the programme and listen to advice but always remember the best guide you will have is your own body.

see

Make sure you visualize your success before you have even taken a physical step towards it. Your mind and body work together as a team and your head is the leader so take time to picture your success right away.

where you won't be disturbed, and to close your eyes. It need only take a couple of minutes and don't be put off if you have never done anything like this before, because it's a straightforward process.

All you have to do is picture yourself looking and feeling good at the start of your cycle ride in 12 weeks' time. You have trained hard and are feeling strong and excited. See yourself zipping along the road smoothly and effortlessly. The kilometres are ticking by and you glide across the line at the end of the race feeling happy. This is a simple exercise, but a good one for gearing you up for your challenge.

How to use your book

Right, now you've pictured the end result in your mind it's time to start taking the steps needed to get there. You won't need to be a rocket scientist to realize that this book is broken down into 12 large steps. Each will include a brief overview of what the focus of that particular week is all about. Read this at the end of the previous week so you've got time to digest it. As with above, visualize the success of the week (come on, you're an old hand at this). Don't skip these few seconds of visualization as they are important in firming up the week ahead in your mind. You will also find snippets of information on things such as food and drink, mental fitness, sleep, and so on, that you can use during your 12 weeks.

The most important page in each section is Your Training Programme and Diary. Again, look over this page at the end of the previous week so the information has plenty of time to sink in. Also ensure you make space in your diary for each day's activity and don't relegate them to, "I'll fit that in somewhere," or you'll get to the end of the day and realize there is no time left. Treat each session as you would an important meeting at work or an appointment with your child's school.

At the bottom of these pages you will also see some traffic lights offering a 'Do This', 'Consider This' and a 'Don't Do This'. These are small tips that you can take on board during the week if you wish. You will also see a 'Reward' on this page, a little something to look forward to when the week is completed. Thoughtful eh? Ah, it's nothing. Use the small notes column to the right of each day to record how you're feeling. It's a great way to end a session and fun to look back on later. You will be amazed at how quickly you progress.

Finally, at the end of each chapter there is a summary of what you have achieved that week. Again, use the notes column to jot down your thoughts and feelings as this will draw a line under the week and help prepare you for the next one. Then it's time for you to give yourself a pat on the back and refer back to your reward.

when

When thinking of taking up an exercise programme for the first time or after an extended break it's important that you check with your doctor that you are fit and healthy enough. Explain your plan and get the thumbs up before starting.

Your aim this week

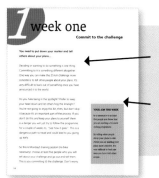

At the end of each week read what's in store for the coming week so you have time to digest it.

This is where you will find a snapshot of your aim for the week. Elsewhere in the section you will find small snippets of information on things such as food and drink or mental fitness.

Training programme

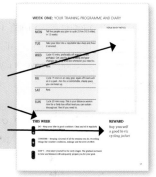

Make sure you diarize your sessions as if they are important appointments. They are.

Use this to jot down your thoughts even if it's just 'Saw Mrs Smith as I set off for my ride. She looked impressed!' or 'Felt great today'.

These are additional tips you can use during your week.

This is what you are looking forward to at the end of the week.

What you have achieved

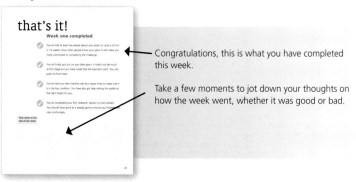

Congratulations, this is what you have completed this week.

Take a few moments to jot down your thoughts on how the week went, whether it was good or bad.

1 week one

Commit to the challenge

You need to put down your marker and tell others about your plans...

Deciding or wanting to do something is one thing. Committing to it is something different altogether. One way you can make this 25 km challenge more concrete is to tell other people about your plans. It's very difficult to back out of something once you have announced it to the world.

Do you hate being in the spotlight? Prefer to keep your head down and let others hog the limelight? You're not going to enjoy this bit, then, but don't skip it because it's an important part of the process. If you don't do this and keep your plans to yourself there is a danger you will just try to follow the programme for a couple of weeks to, "See how it goes". This is a dangerous path to tread and could lead to you giving up early.

So this is Monday's training session (no bike necessary): choose at least five people who you will tell about your challenge and go out and tell them. This is you committing to the challenge. Don't worry,

YOUR AIM THIS WEEK

Is to announce to at least five people you know that you are starting a 12-week cycling programme.

By telling other people about your plans to ride 25 km you are making your plans more concrete. It's very difficult to back out once you have told other people.

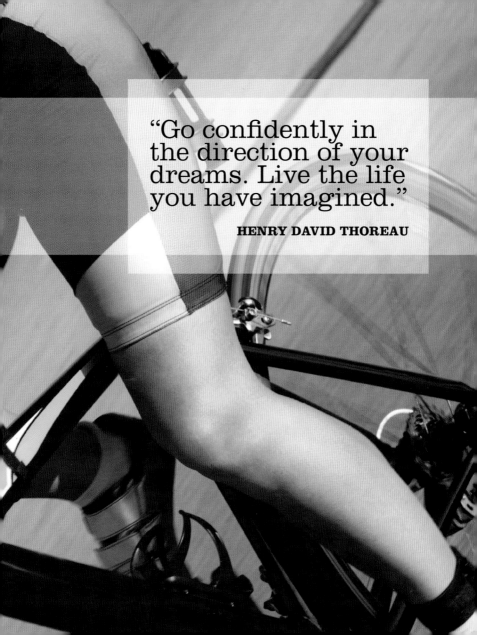

"Go confidently in the direction of your dreams. Live the life you have imagined."

HENRY DAVID THOREAU

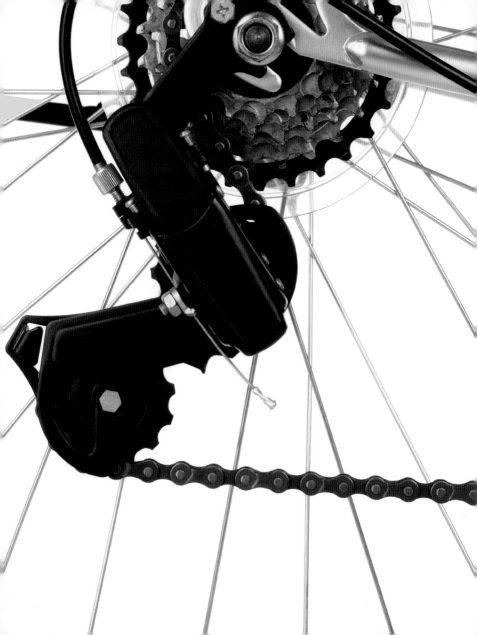

WEEK ONE: YOUR TRAINING PROGRAMME AND DIARY

		YOUR DAILY NOTES
MON	Tell five people you plan to cycle 25 km (15.5 miles). in 12 weeks	
TUE	Take your bike into a reputable bike shop and have it serviced.	
WED	Cycle 15 mins, preferably off-road (in a park perhaps). Get used to the handling and gear changes etc. Stop and rest whenever you need to.	
THU	Rest.	
FRI	Cycle 15 mins in an easy gear, again off-road such as in a park. Aim for a comfortable, steady pace you can keep up.	
SAT	Rest.	
SUN	Cycle 20 mins easy. This is your distance session. Aim for a fairly low effort level you can sustain throughout. Rest if you need to.	

THIS WEEK

 DO – Keep your bike in good condition. Clean and oil it regularly and tighten any loose fittings.

 CONSIDER – Keeping a journal of all the sessions you do, recording things like weather conditions, mileage and the level of effort.

 DON'T – Over-exert yourself in the early stages. The gradual increases in time and distance will adequately prepare you for your goal.

REWARD

Buy yourself a good hi-viz cycling jacket

it's not necessary to burst into the pub and announce to everyone that you have had enough of being out of shape and you'll see them all in 12 weeks looking slim and fit. No-one will believe you anyway if you use this approach.

Keep things casual and work it into the conversation at an appropriate moment. If you get asked what you did on the weekend you can simply reply that you went shopping, bought a book and have decided to start cycling again. Or just leave the book on your desk at work. You'll soon get a few questions about what it is and what your plans are.

People love swapping information (or shall we just call it gossiping?) so be prepared for the news to spread to other people fairly quickly. You'll probably receive a mixed response to your plans. Most people (hopefully) will be supportive but there will be a few who don't seem bothered, or worse still, who put down your idea. Use any negative reactions to make you more determined rather than allowing them to put you off. Negative responses, incidentally, generally come from people who are worried that they could not complete a similar challenge themselves, so allow yourself a wry smile.

But this process should generally be a positive one so make sure at least a few of the people you tell are those you know will back you up – like a best friend.

50

Is the number of minutes you will be exercising this week. This is probably less than the time you might spend having a coffee with a friend or even watching your favourite television programme. Not a lot when you think of it like that is it? Make sure you find the time for exercise just as you would any other activity.

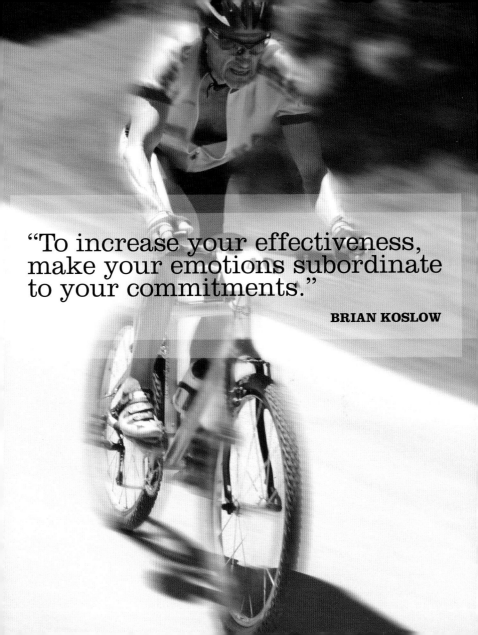

"To increase your effectiveness, make your emotions subordinate to your commitments."

BRIAN KOSLOW

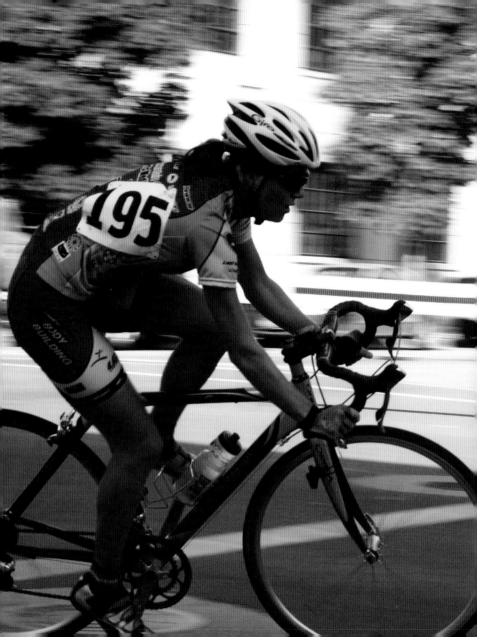

Don't be afraid to use Twitter, Facebook and so on to spread the news if you are feeling confident, but make sure some of this is done face to face as it is more effective.

The rest of the week will be spent shaking off your cycling rustiness. We strongly recommend you get a repair shop to give your bike the once over to make sure everything is still in working order, especially if it has been sitting at the back of the garage for a long time. You could also ask one of the assistants to help you set the saddle at the correct height, a critical element for any cyclist. For the first couple of rides you should find somewhere quiet and safe (like a park), where you can spend a few minutes getting used to the basic handling of the bike again. Even if you consider yourself a good cyclist, it's a good idea to keep away from the pressures of the road while you re-familiarize yourself with two wheels.

Sunday is the day when you will be doing your 'distance' session. Although this is only 20 minutes this week, the time of these rides will gradually be increasing as you get stronger. The most important thing with the Sunday rides is to keep a steady pace so you can complete the session. Try to avoid hills as much as possible at this stage so you can concentrate on building up a nice pedal rhythm with which you feel comfortable. You can start to tackle hills as you get fitter.

Women doing enough exercise

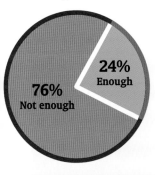

24%
Enough

76%
Not enough

Only 24 per cent of women (37 per cent of men) in the UK do enough exercise according to government health guidelines. Well done, you are on your way to joining the minority!

The figures show just how easy it is for most people to fall into the trap of not keeping fit. Remind yourself of this if you ever feel like giving up in the coming weeks. (1)

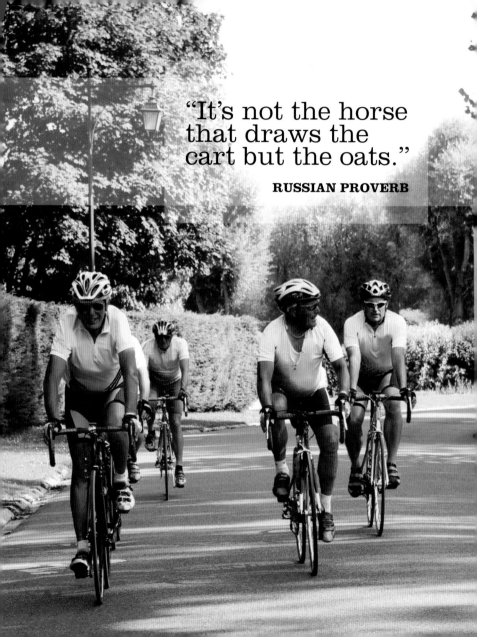

"It's not the horse that draws the cart but the oats."

RUSSIAN PROVERB

that's it!

Week one completed

 You've told at least five people about your plans to cycle a 25 km in 12 weeks. Now other people know your plans it will make you more committed to completing the challenge.

 You've finally got out on your bike again. It might not be much at this stage but you have made that all-important start. You can push on from here.

 You've had your bike checked over by a repair shop to make sure it is in tip-top condition. You have also got help setting the saddle at the right height for you.

 You've completed your first 'distance' session on two wheels. You should have gone at a steady pace to ensure you finished the ride comfortably.

Your notes at the
end of the week

2week two

It's time to hit the road

So far, so good. Now, after the mental preparation, let's get moving…

When you are out of shape and have been away from your bike for a long time, it's important to get mentally prepared before really getting stuck into an exercise programme. That's why most of the work so far has been about getting your mind ready for the weeks ahead, and learning to set aside some time for exercise again. There have also been a couple of sessions on the bike, but this should have been in a safe environment like a park. Now it's time to hit the pedals for real.

There are a few things to consider when you start cycling again after a break of months or years. Firstly, there is no shame in taking breaks every so often at the beginning.

You are only at the start of a 12-week process so remember you need to build up slowly. So although there are some time targets in the programme (eg. aim to cycle for 35 minutes including 15 minutes without stopping on Sunday), do not forget that

YOUR AIM THIS WEEK

Is to get moving – but to always remember to start slowly and maintain an even pace.

It is always better to move towards your end goal by steadily tackling the targets that have been set out in the programme. You should not be afraid to take a break if you need to.

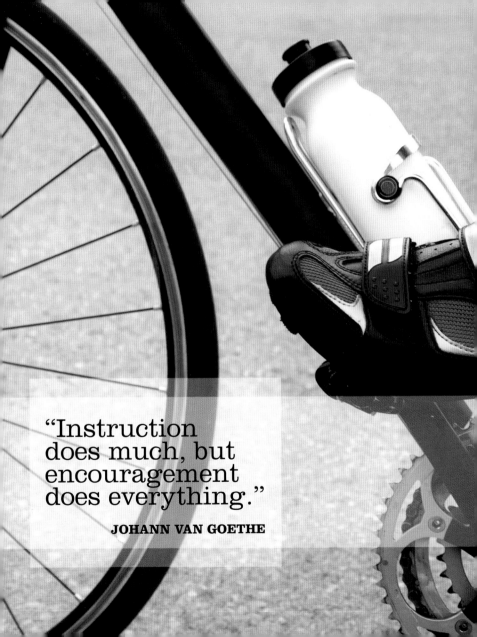

"Instruction
does much, but
encouragement
does everything."

JOHANN VAN GOETHE

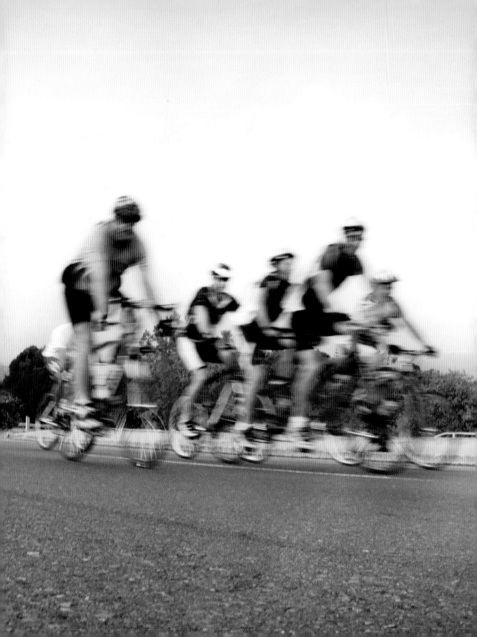

		YOUR DAILY NOTES
MON	Rest.	
TUE	Cycle 25 mins easy. Focus on developing a smooth pedal stroke with a fairly high pedal turnover. Stop whenever you need to.	
WED	Walk 10 mins at a moderate pace.	
THU	Rest.	
FRI	Cycle 20 mins easy. Find a 10 mins lap, away from heavy traffic. Do two laps with a 2 mins rest after the first lap.	
SAT	Rest.	
SUN	Cycle 35 mins easy. Aim to ride for at least 15 mins without stopping.	

THIS WEEK

 DO – Ensure that you have the right size bike frame. A poor fit can cause extreme discomfort and injury.

 CONSIDER – Attending a yoga or T'ai Chi class to learn good breathing and posture.

 DON'T – Try to tackle hilly terrain at this stage. Stay on the flats for now, if you can, and get used to spinning (quick pedal turnover in a relatively easy gear).

REWARD

Treat yourself to a long lie in Sunday morning.

these remain just *targets*, so if you do need to take a break then put it down to the process of building your fitness.

Think back to how you enjoyed being on your bike when you were young: you'd pedal like mad until you were exhausted, stop to get some air and then head off again. Children don't think of it, but stop-start exercise like this is actually an excellent way of building your fitness (although don't do the 'flat-out' thing now!). So rid yourself of the worry about the odd break. Don't use this as an excuse to stop when you like, by the way. You should still *aim* for the targets set down, just worry less about the process of getting there.

The next thing to be aware of is your cycling speed, especially at the start. A good habit to get into is to start slowly, then slow down some more. It's better to ease into your sessions, then build up gently until you have found a nice, comfortable pace that allows you to finish strongly.

Does it really matter what speed you are going at this stage of the programme anyway? After all, anything is faster than when you were slouched in your armchair watching the television. Enjoy being back in the saddle and working your body again. You might be out of breath to start with, and you'll almost certainly feel a bit of stiffness in your legs, but at

2.4 litres

Every day you need to replace 2.4 litres (five pints) of water that is lost or expelled from your body. Although some will come from the food you eat it's important that you drink plenty of water during the day to ensure you do not become dehydrated. (2)

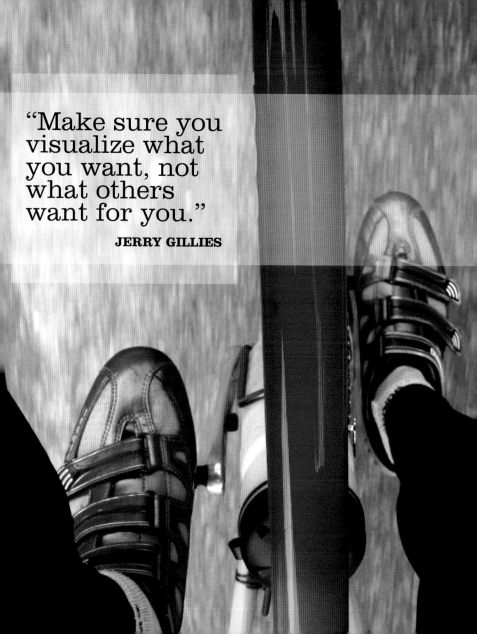

"Make sure you visualize what you want, not what others want for you."

JERRY GILLIES

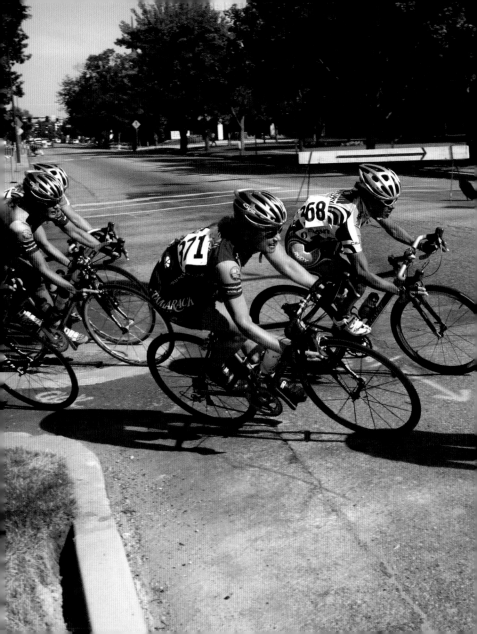

Daily calorie intake

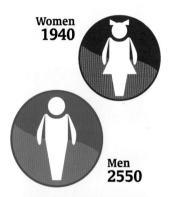

Women
1940

Men
2550

There is no need to get calorie obsessed but nutritional values are clearly marked on most food we buy so it's easy enough to keep an eye on your intake.

What you need per day depends on various factors such as your height, weight and your lifestyle. The chart shows the estimated averages by UK authorities. (3)

least you are on the move again. A bit of stiffness is perfectly natural after exercising, especially when you have been away for so long. Your muscles will adapt and grow in strength quickly, and soon your huffing and puffing days will be behind you.

But, no matter what, always listen to your body. The programme has been carefully planned for a gentle progression towards the end goal – a 25 km cycle ride – but only you will know how much you can manage each day. Alternatively, if you are feeling strong, or particularly enthusiastic, don't do more than what is set out in the programme. It is common at the start of something new like this to get carried away and do too much. But be warned: like the story of the hare and the tortoise, often the people who race off at the beginning are nowhere to be seen at the end. Rather be like the tortoise and complete your challenge.

Finally, are you conscious of how your body looks? If you are you might be worried about how you look when you are cycling. The easy solution to this would be to say, "Don't worry, who cares what other people think anyway?" But, of course, it's not always as easy as that. If this is you, then assuming where you choose to cycle is safe and light, you'll have to use the early mornings and late nights when no one is about or put your bike in the back of your car and drive somewhere where no one will know you.

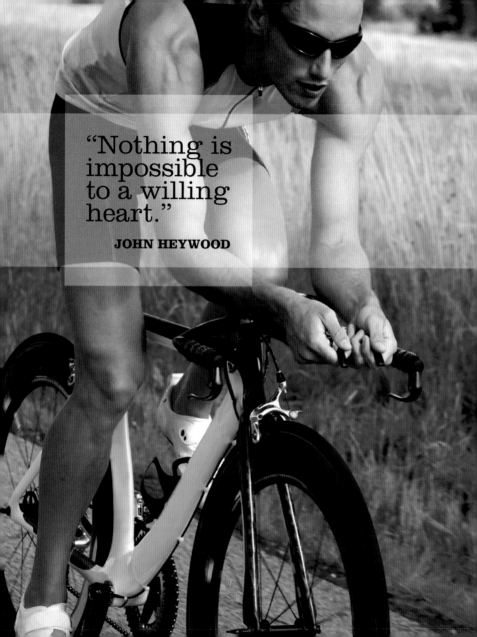

"Nothing is impossible to a willing heart."

JOHN HEYWOOD

that's it!

Week two completed

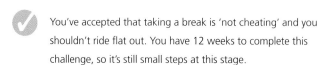

You've accepted that taking a break is 'not cheating' and you shouldn't ride flat out. You have 12 weeks to complete this challenge, so it's still small steps at this stage.

You know to start slowly on your rides and build up to a nice, steady pace.

You can enjoy the fact that you are out exercising again. Even if you are huffing and puffing and experiencing some stiffness in your legs, at least you are back on the move.

You know not to worry about how you look when you cycle. You should not care what other people may think.

Your notes at the end of the week

week three

Rest well and stretch

Get good sleep, stretch often, and treat rest days with respect...

We've already mentioned that your body is good at adapting to change. Granted, it might moan and groan to start with, but it soon takes on more or less whatever you throw at it and deals with it. After all, did it mind when you chose to spend your time relaxing in the armchair with your pizza place's number on speed dial? And now you are exercising, it will deal with that. But there are a few things you can do to help it on its way.

Rest, sleep and stretch. Remember these three things and always consider them as important elements of your programme. In fact, this trinity is every much as important as the actual training sessions.

Firstly rest. When you exercise, you push your body (which is partly why you get stiffness in your muscles), and because of this you need rest to allow your body time to recover. Once it has recovered it will be ready for more exercise, but if you skip the rest (or do not get good rest) then you will feel jaded on your next

YOUR AIM THIS WEEK

Is to treat your rest days as an important part of the programme. Your body needs this time to recover from the workouts.

Within the constraints of your lifestyle, try to spend at least a bit of time getting some quality rest. Set aside time for something you like, such as watching a film or reading.

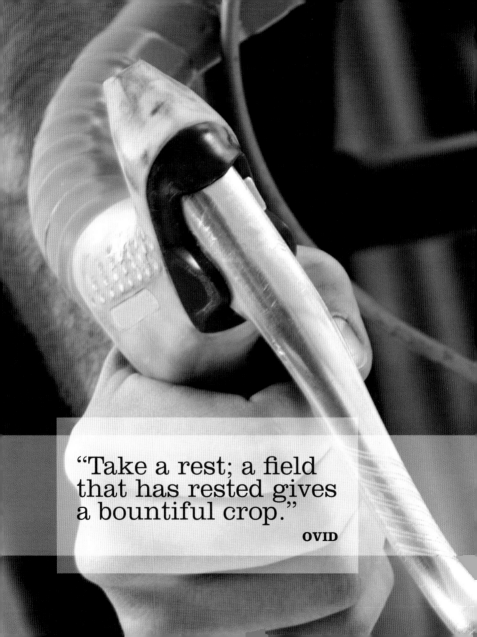

"Take a rest; a field that has rested gives a bountiful crop."

OVID

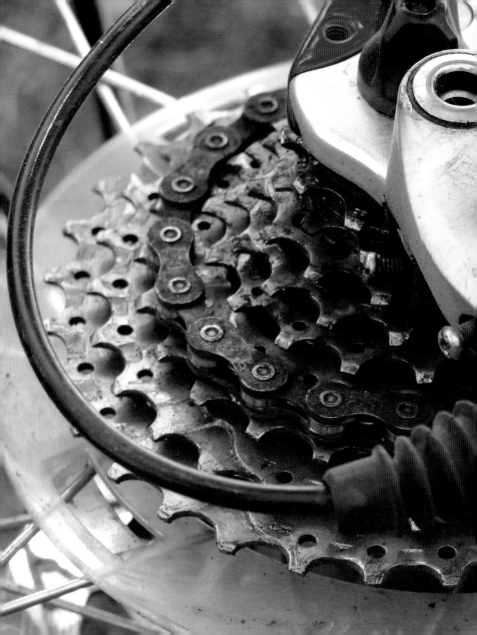

WEEK THREE: YOUR TRAINING PROGRAMME AND DIARY

MON	Rest. This week sees a slight reduction in time, enabling your body to adapt to the exercise and get stronger.
TUE	Cycle 20 mins easy. Warm-up, ride for 8 mins. Focus on a smooth, comfortable stroke and good breathing. Rest for 2 minutes. Repeat x 2.
WED	Walk for 10 mins at a moderate pace.
THU	Rest.
FRI	Cycle 20 mins easy. (Repeat Tuesday's session).
SAT	Rest.
SUN	Cycle 30 mins easy. Try to ride for at least 15 mins without stopping.

THIS WEEK

 DO – Always carry a full bottle of water with you on your bike every time you head out for a ride.

 CONSIDER – Eating more complex carbohydrates, like oats, bread and pasta. These will provide you with the fuel you need to exercise.

 DON'T – Forget to warm-up and cool down. A few minutes light cycling before and after each main set will be adequate.

REWARD

Have a long hot soak with relaxing bath oil.

ride. It sounds straightforward but a lot of people do not get enough quality rest when they are exercising. Do not be one of these people. A rest day is not just the absence of doing exercise, it is actually taking the time to relax your mind and your body.

The reality of modern life means, of course, that you won't be able to sit out in garden dozing in the sun for hours on your rest days. You will have commitments at work, at home, and in your social life, and you can hardly put these on hold for the duration of the programme. What's worse is that the pressures of modern life actually make us feel guilty for resting, because we always feel we should be pushing ourselves to do a bit more (anything will do as long as we are busy). The word 'lazy' seems to be applied to anyone who rests these days. 'March on, march on,' could be the mantra of modern, urban life.

Because of these things, you'll need to fight hard to find time to rest, just as you need to fight hard to find time to exercise. Choose something you enjoy to do, whether it is soaking in a hot bath or watching an inspirational film, and fight to make time for this on your rest days.

Needless to say, if quality rest is good, then quality sleep is even better. Most of us grow up hearing that eight hours a night is the 'correct' amount of sleep for an adult. However, everybody is different. You

38%

Unless you're a particular fan of hospital food, being inactive doesn't really hold much appeal. UK research has found that inactive people spend 38 per cent more days in hospital than active people, visit their doctor 5.5 per cent more and use specialist services 13 per cent more. (4)

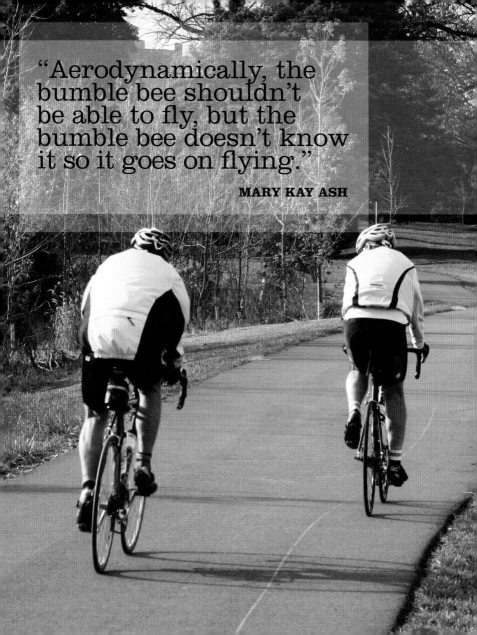

"Aerodynamically, the bumble bee shouldn't be able to fly, but the bumble bee doesn't know it so it goes on flying."

MARY KAY ASH

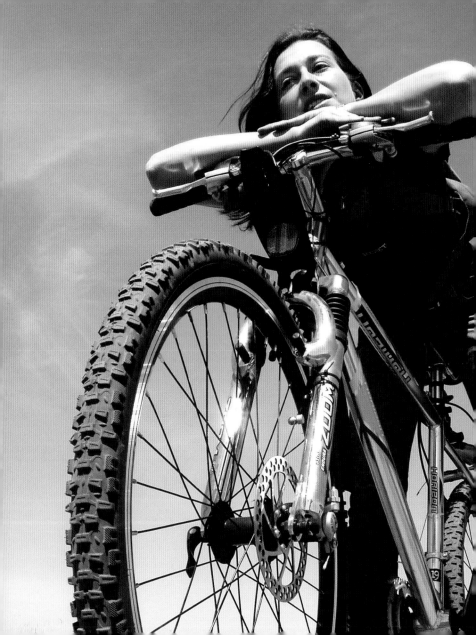

may need a bit more sleep than eight hours, or you may be happy with less. Again, listen to your body, as only you will know what the right amount is for you.

Try to get into a regular sleep pattern throughout the whole week. A lot of people skip sleep during the week (oh, those pressures of work and partying again), then 'catch up' by sleeping in on the weekend (young children permitting). However, your body adapts best when it gets into a regular sleep routine, so as much as your lifestyle permits, try to get to bed at the same time every night and wake at the same time every morning.

Stretching is something that is often overlooked as the 'soft' part of exercising. You've spent all that time on the armchair and now, after finally rousing yourself, you just want to get on with it. This is a perfectly natural reaction. But give your poor old muscles a break before you start hammering them on the pedals. Always make time, a few minutes will do, stretching out every part of your body, paying particular attention to your legs and back, both before and after a training session. In the early days you may even feel yourself stiffening up during a ride (probably around your neck and shoulders). This is because you are tensing up too much. If this happens, stop and stretch out these muscles again. Stretching is also something we would recommend you do on your rest days to keep your muscles loose.

Calories in takeaways

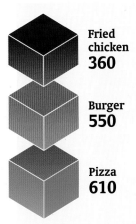

**Fried
chicken
360**

**Burger
550**

**Pizza
610**

Nothing beats a tasty takeaway, but keep an eye on the calories. The chart above refers to a Big Mac (215 g, 7.6 oz), a Pizza Hut Pepperoni 6-inch (15 cm) Personal Pan Pizza, a KFC chicken breast (163 g, 5.8 oz). (5)

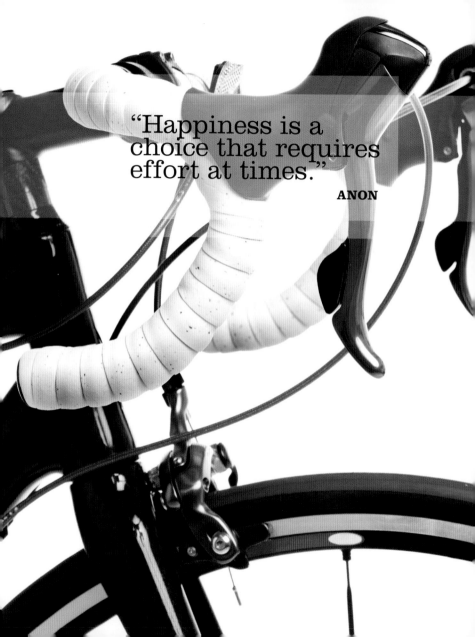

"Happiness is a choice that requires effort at times."

ANON

that's it!

Week three completed

 You are giving the rest days the importance they deserve. Your body will use this rest time to rebuild the muscles that have been worked during your cycle rides.

 You know the best rest you can get is sleep. Try to settle into a regular sleep pattern rather than trying to 'catch up' when you are exhausted.

 You know it is important to warm-up your body in preparation for a session, and to cool down afterwards.

 You want to keep loose for your sessions, so you will consider doing a bit of stretching on your rest days.

Your notes at the end of the week

week four

Make cycling a habit

Before you know it cycling will be an integral part of your life…

When the pressures of life (particularly the pressures of time) got the best of you one day in the not so distant past, you decided you were going to go straight home, order a pizza and lounge in front of the television. It was nice, just what you needed after a tough day at work. So you did it again.

Over the next few weeks you did it again and again. Then, you, your armchair and the pizza delivery man became very good friends. The whole thing had become a habit you didn't ask for and probably never wanted. But once you engrain something as a habit it's pretty hard to shift, so you continued with the pizza-television-armchair thing.

Well, here's the good news. Just as you formed that bad habit by repeating the action over and over again, so you can form the good habit of exercising in the same way. Bad habits, good habits, they work just the same. So stick to the programme, and keep exercising hard in the knowledge you are gradually

YOUR AIM THIS WEEK

Is to recognize that good habits are formed in exactly the same way as bad habits. You simply keep repeating the same action over and over again.

So for you to make cycling a habit, all you have to do is keep going with the programme – it's as simple as that.

"Cultivate only the habits you are willing should master you."

ELBERT HUBBARD

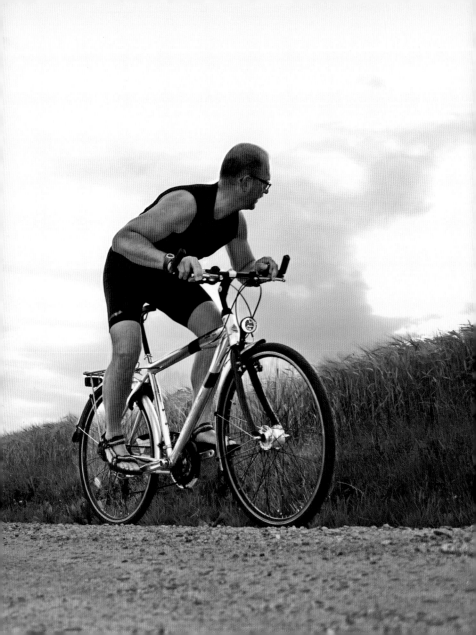

WEEK FOUR: YOUR TRAINING PROGRAMME AND DIARY

MON	Rest. This week sees the inclusion of an optional cross-training session on Thursday and Saturday (eg. swimming or gym). Take it easy.
TUE	Cycle 30 mins easy. Warm-up, ride 8 mins. Focus on a smooth, comfortable stroke and good breathing. Rest for 2 mins. Repeat x 3.
WED	Walk for 12 minutes at a moderate pace.
THU	Rest or cross train. Do something fun.
FRI	Cycle 30 minutes easy. Warm-up, ride 6 mins at a comfortable pace. Increase effort level slightly for last 30 secs. Spin or rest for 2 mins. Repeat x 3.
SAT	Rest or cross train.
SUN	Cycle 40 mins easy. Try to ride for at least 30 minutes without stopping.

THIS WEEK

 DO – Practise a smooth pedal stroke with a fairly high turnover as this is more efficient. Always use the ball of you feet to push down on the pedals.

 CONSIDER – Learning how to fix punctures! If you're now sure how to, ask in your local bike shop or read a manual.

 DON'T – Force yourself to go out if you have a cold or other illness. There is nothing to be gained from this from a fitness point of view, and you could endanger your health.

REWARD

Treat yourself to a massage.

forming a good habit that you actually want in your life. Before you know it you will be waking up, pulling on your cycling gear and heading out the door for your ride without even thinking about it. "Hang on, how did that happen?" you might ask yourself. It will happen because you will keep at it.

So what can you do to help this process along? The first thing is to continue to jealously guard your training sessions and not let anything (within reason) get in their way.

You should continue to mark down the training sessions in your diary or on your phone as if they are important appointments. Consider looking ahead and punching in all the sessions right up to the end so you can plan ahead with things like holidays and long-term commitments. Remember, the programme has been devised for people with busy lives, so it is flexible if you need to swap one or two days. If, because you have a work or family emergency to attend to, you may have to miss a session. Sometimes this is unavoidable, so don't beat yourself up. Sort out what needs sorting out and return to the programme at the next available opportunity.

A good way to stick to the programme is to train with someone else. Find a training buddy who has more or less the same level of fitness as you. Of course, it would be a lot more fun if you are both

66days

It takes an average of 66 days to form a habit. Although this is the average time it takes to turn something new into automatic behaviour a habit can form quicker for some or take considerably longer for others – so stick at it and exercise will soon become a habit for you. (6)

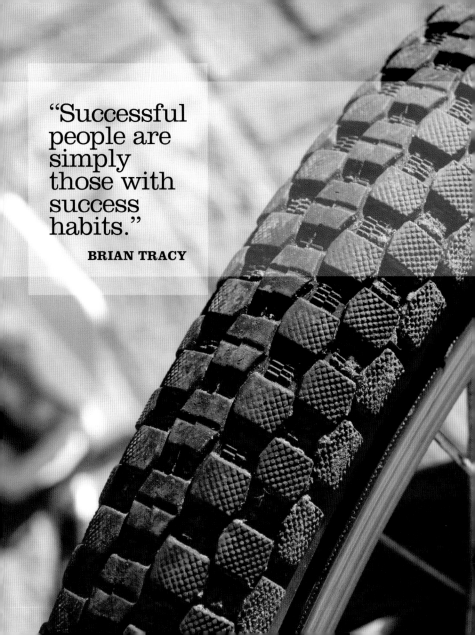

"Successful people are simply those with success habits."

BRIAN TRACY

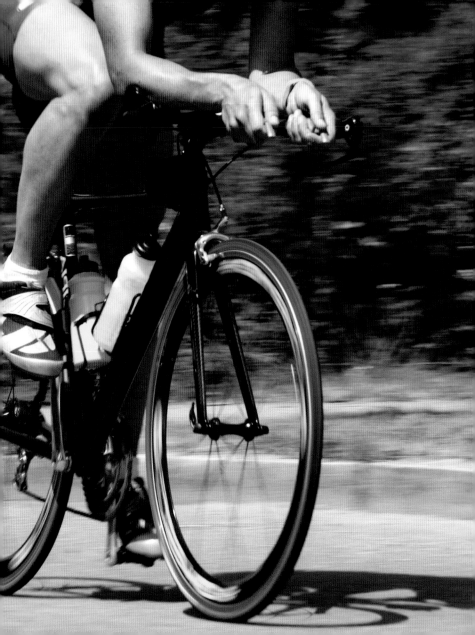

How many people get enough sleep?

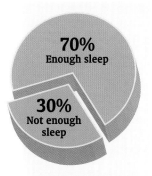

70%
Enough sleep

30%
Not enough sleep

Thirty per cent of working adults do not sleep enough (defined as less than six hours on average per day) according to a US survey.

A lack of sleep is associated with various health problems and makes it particularly difficult to train hard and get fit so make sure your lifestyle allows you to be part of the 70 per cent. (7)

follow the whole cycling programme together, but this doesn't have to be the case. Maybe there is a friend who would like to join on the distance rides on Sundays, and someone else who joins you for the walks, for instance.

The best thing about having a training buddy is that you both help each other along. When you not feeling motivated, a kind word from your buddy can help lift you, and vice versa. It's also very difficult to skip a training session when you know your buddy is waiting for you. Ask around, you will be surprised at how many of your friends and family will be interested in joining you, even for just a part of your training.

It's also a good idea to do your training at a time of day you are least likely to be disturbed. There is no point planning to ride in the mornings if you know you have children to get ready for school, then head off for work yourself (unless you don't mind getting up *really* early).

Again, remember to remain flexible for things that may crop up in your life. If you decide the best time for you to train is in the evenings when the rest of the family is in front of the television, don't be afraid to swap to a lunchtime session if a friend's party comes up. Exercising should be a fun part of your life, but it can also fit in with the rest of the things you want and like to do.

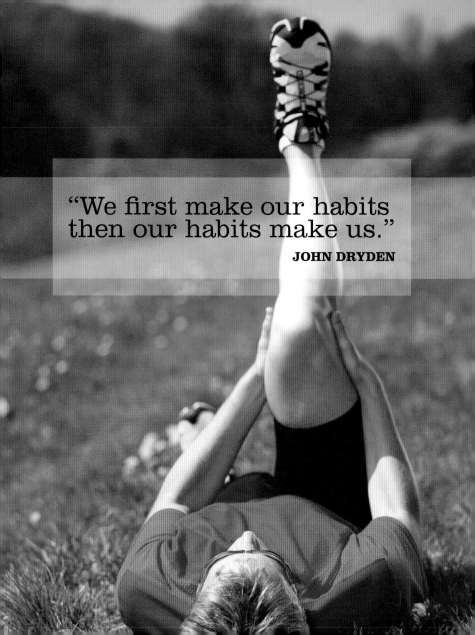

"We first make our habits
then our habits make us."

JOHN DRYDEN

that's it!

Week four completed

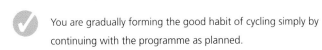 You are gradually forming the good habit of cycling simply by continuing with the programme as planned.

You know that good and bad habits work in exactly the same way. If you repeat an action often enough – such as cycling regularly – then you will form the habit.

You are treating your training sessions as important appointments. Apart from emergencies you should not let anything get in the way of your training.

You should train at a time of day when you are least likely to be disturbed but remain flexible.

Your notes at the
end of the week

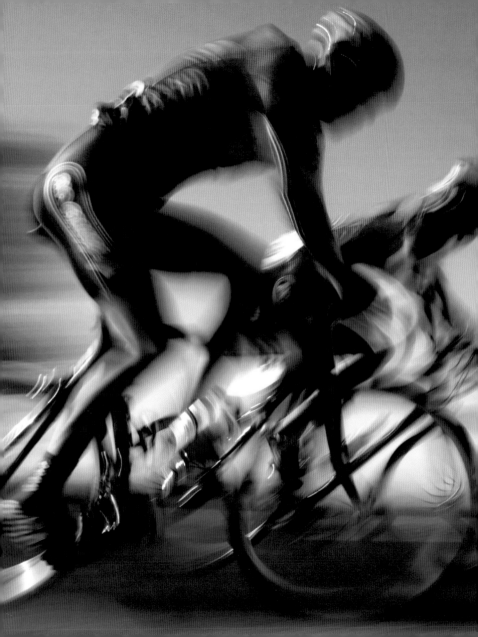

week five

Enjoy the smoothness of cycling

Concentrate on a smooth pedal stroke to fully enjoy cycling…

One of the most amazing feelings for a cyclist is when everything clicks into place. Your shoulders feel nice and relaxed, your legs spin effortlessly, and the bike is speeding along the tarmac for fun. Let's complete the picture with the sun in the sky and a nice cool breeze on your face. Sometimes, when out on a bike, especially when there is no traffic about, life certainly can feel sweet.

Even though you have only had a few sessions so far, hopefully you have already had a taste of that great feeling (even if it has just been on the downhills!). The good news is that the more you cycle, the more you ease that rustiness out of your limbs, and the more you can enjoy that smooth feeling when everything clicks into place. You can help with this by spending a bit of time looking at your cycling technique

The main thing to concentrate on is to maintain a smooth pedal stroke and avoid that jerking

YOUR AIM THIS WEEK

Is to work on developing a smooth pedal stroke when you are turning the pedals.

It is not necessary to get caught up in the technical and scientific details of technique at this stage. Concentrate on keeping the pedals moving at an even pace so the movement feels smooth rather than as if you are fighting your bike.

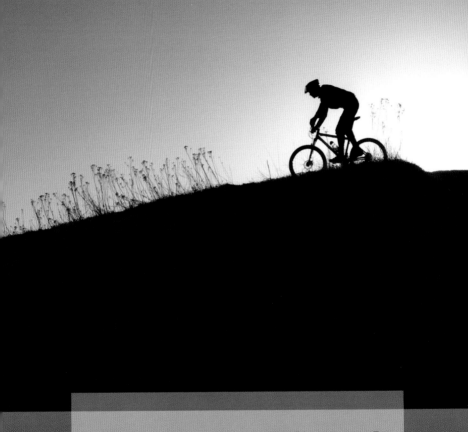

"Success is a welcomed gift for the uninhibited mind."

ADLIN SINCLAIR

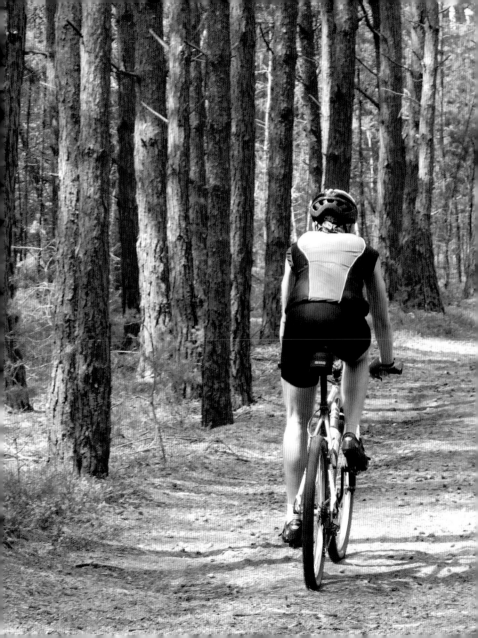

		YOUR DAILY NOTES
MON	Rest.	
TUE	Cycle 35 mins easy. Warm-up, ride 12 mins. Focus on a smooth, comfortable stroke. Rest or spin for 2 mins. Repeat x 2.	
WED	Walk 12 mins at a moderate pace.	
THU	Rest or cross train.	
FRI	Cycle 35 mins easy. Warm-up, ride 8 mins at a comfortable pace. Increase effort level slightly for last 30 secs. Spin or rest for 2 mins. Repeat x 3.	
SAT	Rest.	
SUN	Cycle 45 mins easy. Try to ride for at least 30 mins without stopping.	

THIS WEEK

 DO – Aim to get more sleep as the sessions increase. Sleep enhances all areas of growth and will improve your performance.

 CONSIDER – Drinking more water throughout the day. Aim to drink a glass after each meal, and carry a bottle on your bike, especially in hot weather.

 DON'T – Give up! You're almost at the halfway stage now. The long term benefits from regular exercise are well worth the effort.

REWARD

Switch off your phone for an hour, put your feet up and relax.

movement as your legs turn the pedals. This is due to what is known as the 'dead spots' at the top and the bottom of the pedal stroke. It is important to maintain an even force (as is possible) on each turn when both pushing down (remember to use the ball of your feet) and pulling up the pedals. The more efficient you are with this movement the less energy you will use, and the more you will get out of each pedal stroke.

Professional cyclists spend years analyzing their pedal stroke for efficiency but you've only got 12 weeks so concentrate on feeling a comfortable rhythm during the full turn. If you spend a bit of time consciously thinking about it now, it will become second nature to you very soon.

You should also concentrate on keeping loose and relaxed over the handlebars. It is easy to tense up if you grip too tight and this tensing will spread. If you feel this happening simply breathe out deeply a couple of times and you will feel the looseness coming back to your body. If necessary, stop cycling altogether, shake out your limbs one by one and give your neck and shoulders a gentle roll.

If you haven't already done so, this is the time to buy some proper cycling kit. You can train for and ride 25 km with any old pair of shorts or leggings and a baggy T-shirt if you really want to. However,

30mins

When running at a pace of 8 kph (5 mph) for 30 minutes a person weighing 56 kg (125 pounds) will burn 240 calories, while for someone weighing 70 kg (155 pounds) it is 298 calories, and at 84 kg (185 pounds) it is 355 calories. Figures are the same for circuit training, while swimming breaststroke burns 300, 372 and 444 calories respectively. For cycling at 19-22 kph (12-14 mph) the calories burnt are 240, 298 and 355. [8]

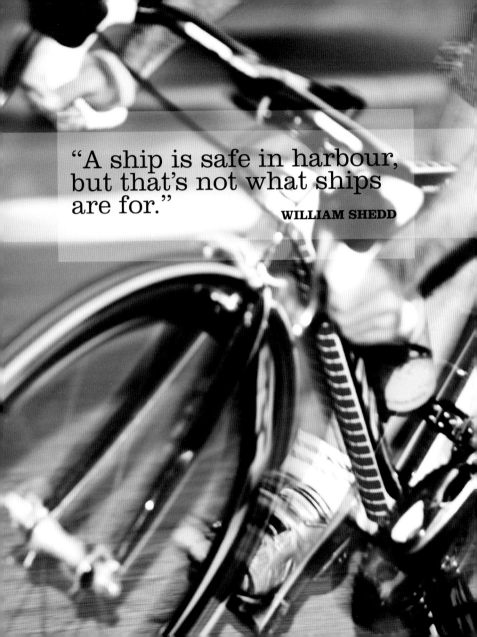

"A ship is safe in harbour, but that's not what ships are for."

WILLIAM SHEDD

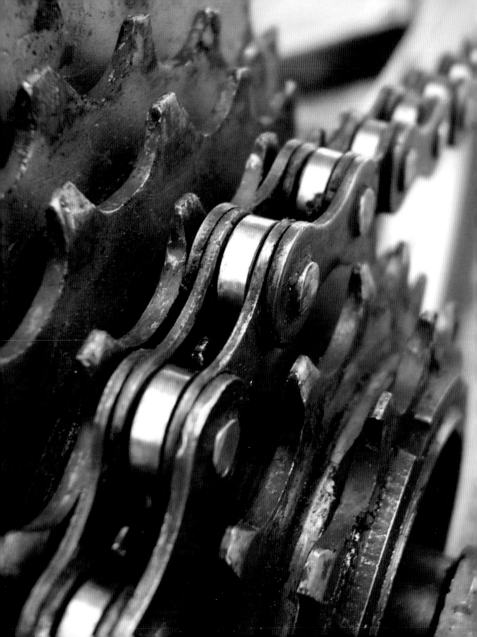

Calories in drinks

Calories (per 100 ml, 3.4 fl oz)

Whole milk	**63**
Cola	**37**
Cappuccino	**30**
Water	**0**

It's easy to rack up the calories you consume in drinks each day. Don't cut back and become dehydrated, just balance the type of drinks you enjoy. The chart shows figures for a glass of milk, Coca-Cola and a Starbucks cappuccino with whole milk. (9)

built-for-purpose cycling kit is padded in the right places (around your bum) and designed using breathable material that operates better in different weather conditions. Do you prefer a sore backside and a wet, soggy T-shirt clinging to your body, or cycling kit that reduces rubbing and absorbs a minimal amount of rain?

You should always carry a wind jacket, which you can put on if the temperature drops or the rain clouds decide to empty. And if you are lucky enough to live in a hot and sunny climate, do not forget your sun cream.

If you are feeling particularly keen you may have considered buying some proper cycling cleats. Think long and hard before you do, as these take some getting used to and you have enough on your cycling plate at the moment. You should, however, make sure the sports shoes you use are as rigid as possible (beachwear is not good if you haven't guessed already) to ensure you don't lose efficiency in your pedal stroke and get a foot injury.

It's also worth looking at getting a decent saddle for the same reason, as you'll want cycling shorts with similar protection (ie. it's more comfortable for your backside). Although certain saddles are more for touring than racing, let's go for comfort rather than speed at this stage.

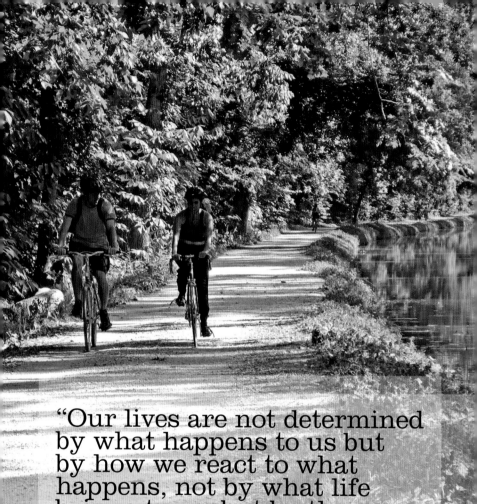

"Our lives are not determined by what happens to us but by how we react to what happens, not by what life brings to us, but by the attitude we bring to life."

ANON

that's it!

Week five completed

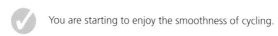

✓ You are starting to enjoy the smoothness of cycling.

✓ You know to keep loose and relaxed over the handlebars. Don't be afraid to stop and shake out the stiffness if need be.

✓ You know the best way thing you can do to improve your cycling technique is to concentrate on maintaining a smooth pedal stroke and avoid that inefficient jerking stroke.

✓ You should have bought some proper cycling kit and a padded saddle. The correct equipment will help you cycle better, feel better and it will help you avoid soreness.

Your notes at the end of the week

week six

Fitness benefits are coming

Trust your subconscious. It will work to give you plenty of benefits from your training…

Your mind is a remarkably powerful tool. This is why we encouraged you to visualize your success right at the start (and why we will continue to encourage you to do so in the future).

While your body moans and groans that it can't go any further, grumbles for food that will do it no good at all, and complains at the first sign of discomfort, your mind knows better. It has been hardwired to understand what you body can achieve if it is pushed correctly, and how it can get it there.

You already released the power of your subconscious when you set the goal to ride 25 km in 12 weeks. Since then your subconscious has been hard at work attracting things to support the goal, even if you have not noticed it yet. As you continue with your training, and maintain your focus on the 25 km target, you may find yourself drawn to new strategies relating to nutrition, kit, or cycling techniques and so on. So while you may not have

YOUR AIM THIS WEEK

Is to relax and let your subconscious get to work. It's a powerful tool and you released it when you set your goal to ride 25 km.

As you continue with the training programme and your body gets fitter, your subconscious will be busy attracting other positives, such as healthier eating and so on.

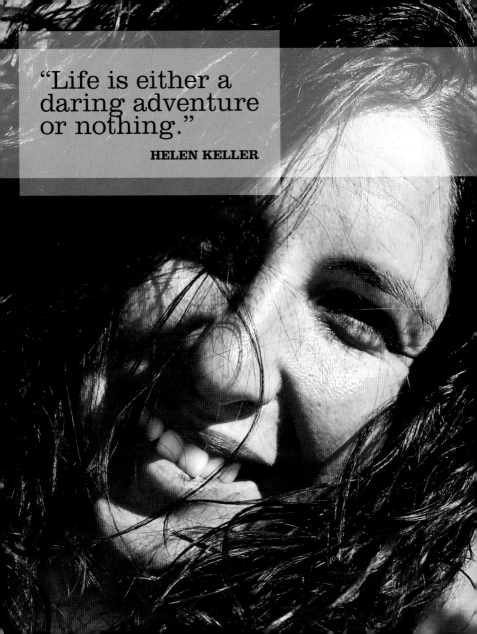

"Life is either a daring adventure or nothing."

HELEN KELLER

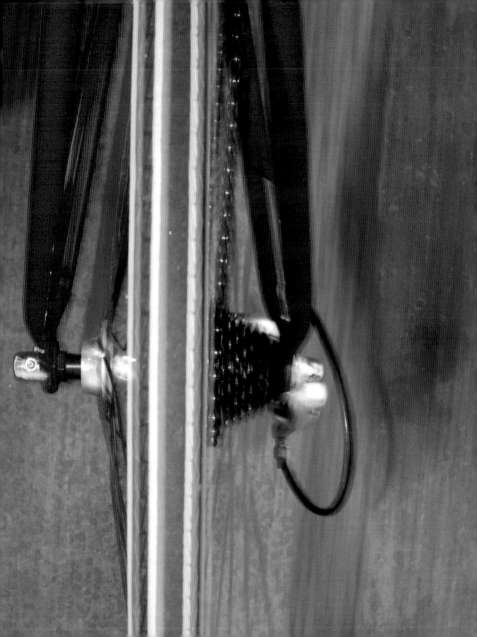

		YOUR DAILY NOTES
MON	Rest.	
TUE	Cycle 30 mins easy. Warm-up, ride for 12 mins. Focus on a smooth, comfortable stroke. Rest or spin for 2 mins. Repeat x 2.	
WED	Walk 10 mins at a moderate pace.	
THU	Rest or cross train.	
FRI	Cycle 30 mins easy. Warm-up, ride for 6 mins at a comfortable pace. Increase effort level slightly for last 30 secs. Spin or rest for 2 mins. Repeat x 3.	
SAT	Rest or cross train.	
SUN	Cycle 40 mins easy. Try to ride the full distance out and back.	

THIS WEEK

DO – Notice the slight reductions in certain weeks. This allows both mind and body to adapt, ready for the next stage.

CONSIDER – Reviewing your performance so far. What do you consider your weakness? Which areas could you improve?

DON'T – Obsess about your goal. Take each stage as it comes and focus on the objectives set out in your programme.

REWARD

A takeaway of your choice to celebrate your achievement so far.

the slightest bit of interest in nutrition you may suddenly find yourself eating more healthily as your subconscious works to replenish your body with what it needs for its training. Or, after a few sore backside moments (because you persist in wearing those baggy board shorts on the distance rides), you could find yourself popping into a cycling shop to get those padded shorts. It sounds simple enough, but this is your subconscious at work.

But don't worry about these 'other' things. You've already taken the important step of deciding to start exercising, and you are still following this programme. It's not necessary to change other things in your life, as we stressed at the start. The other positives – better diet, improved cycling technique, and so on – will follow in due course.

Who knows, maybe you have already noticed yourself piling an extra spoonful of vegetables on to your plate once in a while? Just remember, no one is expecting you to become a fitness fanatic overnight, so simply keep focused on your training and let the other good stuff happen in its own time.

This is also the time to start planning the details for the day of your 25 km ride. Although there are still a few weeks to go in the programme, if you haven't already done so, this is now the time to start thinking about where you will complete your challenge.

5days

Now you have started exercising you are well on your way to meeting guidelines set out by many government health experts – adults aged over 18 should exercise at moderate intensity for 30 minutes at least five days per week. The exercise does not need to be consecutive but should be in bouts of at least 10 minutes at a time. (10)

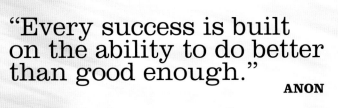

"Every success is built on the ability to do better than good enough."

ANON

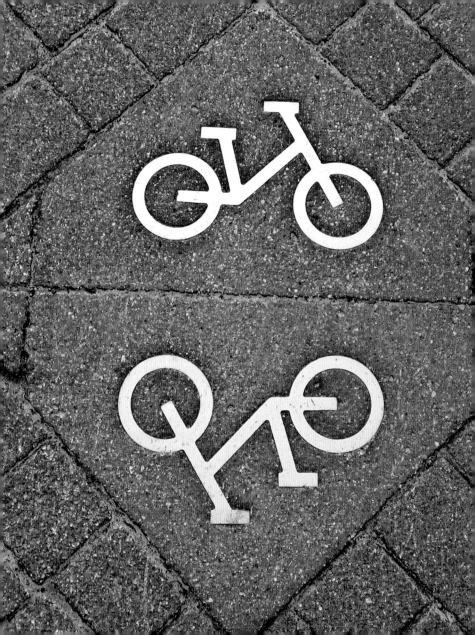

Calories burnt in 30 mins

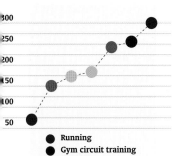

300
250
200
150
100
50

- ● Running
- ● Gym circuit training
- ● Swimming
- ○ Cycling
- ● Mowing the lawn
- ◉ Walking
- ● Ironing

Different activities use up varying amounts of energy and it's worth noting that even some daily activities help keep you healthy.

The chart shows figures for a walking lawn mower, brisk walking at 6.5 kph (4 mph), moderate cycling at 19-22 kph (12-14 mph), swimming at a pace of 46 metres (50 yards) a minute, and running at 9.5 kph (6 mph). (11)

Certainly the best thing to do, and the most fun, would be to identify an organized cycling race that coincides with your target date and enter it. Unfortunately, unlike a sport such as running, there is not a glut of races for casual or novice cyclists. There are, however, a few races out there if you search hard enough, so you may find something that fits the bill.

Don't worry if the race is a fair distance away from where you live. Simply turn your challenge into a weekend away. Grab your partner, family or friends (or all of them!) and plan to head off. This will also help to keep you motivated in the coming weeks. Entering an organized race gives you the added benefit of support, with water stations, marshals for road safety and, of course, the distance has been measured out exactly. You could also keep your eyes open for sponsored rides put together by a school or another community organization.

If, however, you do draw a blank with your search for a race, or just prefer to keep this as a solo exercise, there is no problem in organizing your own 'race' for your challenge. It's easy enough to measure out your own 25 km route by car in advance, then come 'race day' it's down to you, your legs and a stopwatch. Remember to choose a course that is safe and free of heavy traffic. Also try to make your 'race' route different from your usual training routes to keep it special.

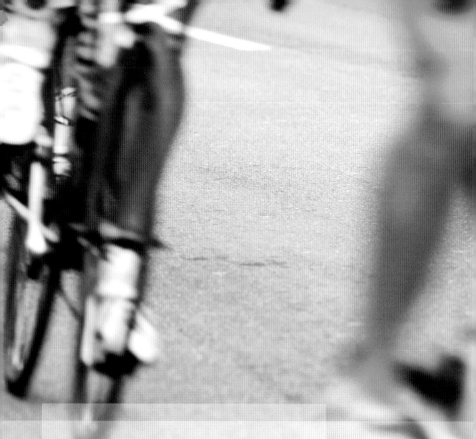

"Health is the thing that makes you feel that now is the best time of the year."

FRANKLIN P ADAMS

that's it!

Week six completed

 You released the power of your subconscious when your set your 25 km goal. It will now work with your body to achieve that goal.

 You know various benefits – such as healthier eating – will follow as you continue training.

 You know that these benefits will come naturally and you should not force them. Keep your focus on the end goal of the 25 km ride. Trust your subconscious to sort things out and enjoy the benefits when they arrive.

 You have started thinking about the details for the day of your challenge. It will bring everything into focus once you know where and when you will be riding.

Your notes at the end of the week

week seven

You're well on your way

Think back and congratulate yourself on how far you have come already...

Keeping your mind positive is important, especially now you are so far into the training programme. Be proud of what you have achieved already. Worry less about the training days when you struggle, and focus and repeat what you did on the good days. Your memory should be short for failures and long for successes (this incidentally is a good rule to apply in other areas of your life as well).

It's inevitable there will be some days when you don't feel like training. Even if you've done everything right: kept hydrated, slept and eaten well, stretched out your muscles, some days you just don't 'feel right' (not in the ill sense). Don't worry about these, just accept they are part and parcel of the whole picture. Concentrate on the positives you get from them – you've worked a few more kilometres into your legs and maybe fine-tuned your technique a bit more.

Remember to keep thinking of the programme as a series of small building blocks which you are piecing

YOUR AIM THIS WEEK

Is to keep focused on your good training days and tuck the bad ones away in your short-term memory.

Accept there are some days when you just don't feel like training or don't 'feel right'. Even on these days you are still adding another block as you build towards your end goal.

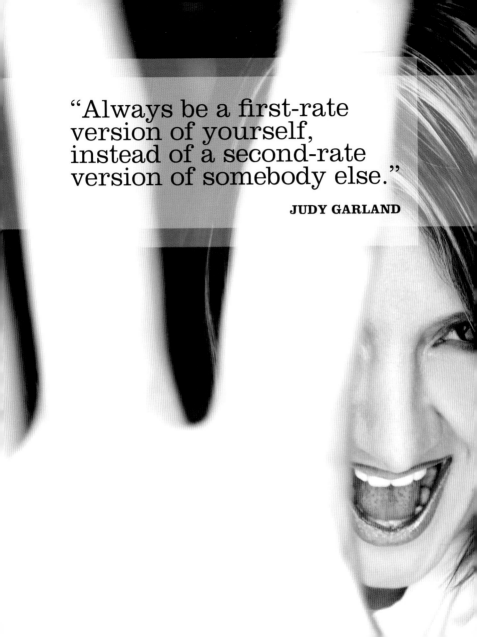

"Always be a first-rate version of yourself, instead of a second-rate version of somebody else."

JUDY GARLAND

WEEK SEVEN: YOUR TRAINING PROGRAMME AND DIARY

		YOUR DAILY NOTES
MON	Rest. This week includes some hill work, so rest as much as you can in between.	
TUE	Cycle 40 mins easy-moderate. Find a fairly hilly area, away from traffic. Warm-up, ride for 10 mins (include at least one hill). Rest or spin for 2 mins. Repeat x 3.	
WED	Walk for 14 mins at a moderate pace.	
THU	Rest or cross train.	
FRI	Cycle 40 mins easy-moderate. Warm-up, ride for 15 mins. Increase effort level for 30 secs every 5 mins. Rest or spin for 2 mins. Repeat x 2.	
SAT	Rest or cross train.	
SUN	Cycle 50 mins easy. Try to ride the full distance out and back.	

THIS WEEK

 DO – Reduce the volume of exercise if you feel it is too much. Listen to your body and include an extra day's rest if you feel it would help.

 CONSIDER – Joining a local cycling club. You may well benefit from the support and encouragement of other cyclists.

 DON'T – Get involved in racing others at this stage. Stick to your programme and look for small but lasting improvements.

REWARD

One big bar of chocolate, all to yourself!

together. Bit by bit the blocks will build towards your end goal – the 25 km cycle ride. So even on those days you don't 'feel right', you can at least console yourself that you have built another important block.

By exercising regularly you are slowly sharpening not only your body but also your mind. If you need reminding of this look no further than your own notes (you have been keeping notes haven't you?).

In the early days it is likely the pages were littered with comments such as, "I was exhausted after a few minutes, will I even make it?" Compare these early comments to the ones you are writing down now to see just how far you have come in so short a time. Again, concentrate on the positive days and let those inspire you. Always think of those good days when everything clicked into place and your training ride felt like a breeze.

You are now well into the programme (in fact, at the start of this week you are at the halfway stage). If you have stuck to the programme rigidly then you will have done 18 cycle rides, five walks, plus a few cross training sessions (and hopefully plenty of stretching) to date. This forms a decent amount of work and will form the base for what is follow as you push on to the end goal. We remind you of this because it is not uncommon at this stage for some people to worry they have not done enough work. This is mainly

7, 8, 9

Most of us grow up being told that we need a 'good eight hours sleep' every night. Experts recommend seven to nine hours sleep a night for an adult – only you will know what is right for you. Try to get into a regular sleep pattern instead of trying to 'catch up' on the weekends as this re-sets your sleep cycle. (12)

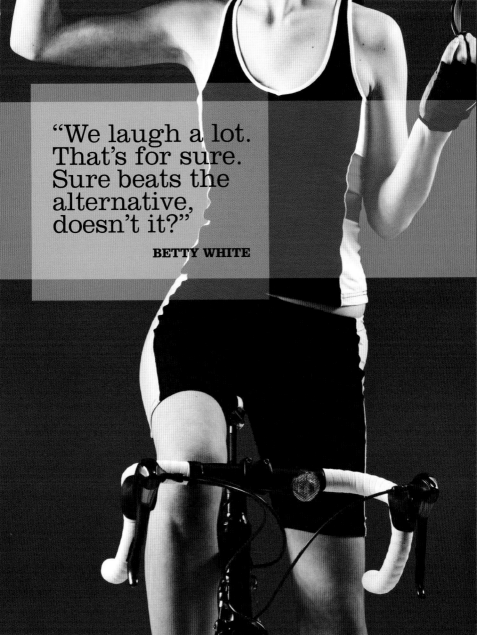

"We laugh a lot. That's for sure. Sure beats the alternative, doesn't it?"

BETTY WHITE

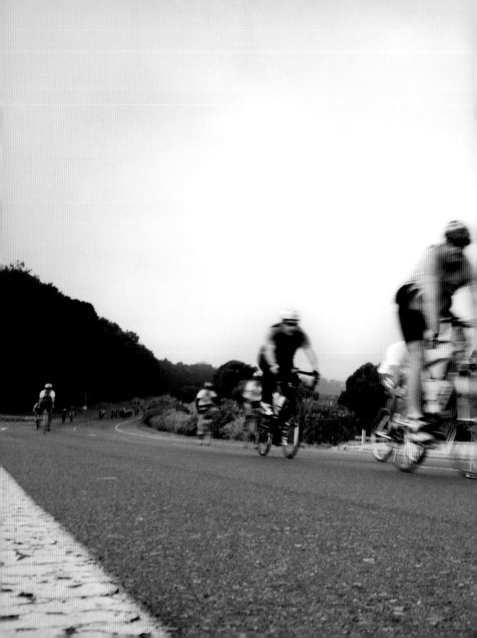

because the end is now in sight (it was so far away at the start it didn't feel real). The trouble with worrying you have not done enough work is that you are tempted to do extra. This can be extra sessions (when you should be resting) or doing more distance/time than what is set out in the training programme.

This is to be avoided at all costs. The programme has been carefully designed to ease you gently from the armchair to a 25 km ride in 12 weeks. Trust in it to get you there. By doing more, you are harming your chances of finishing by exhausting yourself.

How about focusing your energy on something more positive instead? Maybe you could use your challenge to raise some money for charity? Of course, if you did find a sponsored ride to enter then that makes things simple, but even if you are organizing your own 'race' day there is no reason why you can't still raise some money for charity. Most of us have a charity that is close to our heart for personal reasons, and signing up can help give you an added incentive to complete what you have set out to do. Charities will be happy to receive your support, so fire off an e-mail and explain what you are planning to do. Most charities are geared up for this and will have special packs with everything you'll need to raise money, such as sponsorship forms, posters and so on. There are also online sites where you can set up your challenge and people are able to donate money.

Health benefits of fitness

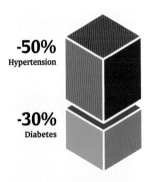

-50%
Hypertension

-30%
Diabetes

Exercising regularly reduces your risk of contracting many chronic diseases. These include Hypertension (50%), Ischaemic heart disease (40%), breast cancer (27%), a stroke (27%). (13)

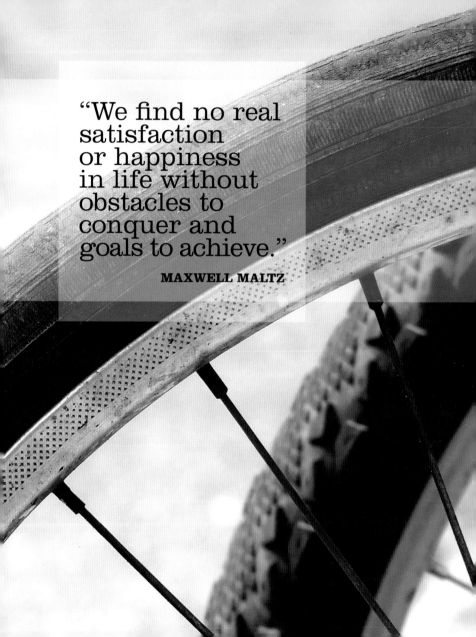

"We find no real satisfaction or happiness in life without obstacles to conquer and goals to achieve."

MAXWELL MALTZ

that's it!

Week seven completed

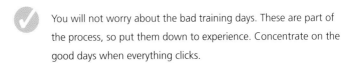 You will not worry about the bad training days. These are part of the process, so put them down to experience. Concentrate on the good days when everything clicks.

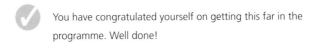 You have congratulated yourself on getting this far in the programme. Well done!

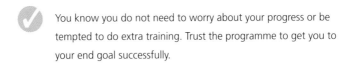 You know you do not need to worry about your progress or be tempted to do extra training. Trust the programme to get you to your end goal successfully.

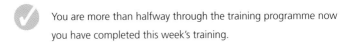 You are more than halfway through the training programme now you have completed this week's training.

Your notes at the end of the week

8 week eight

Picture your success

Look ahead to your 25 km ride and see yourself completing it in style…

The short visualization exercise you did at the start of the programme was all about tuning your mind into what you wished to achieve. It's a great exercise because your mind works with your body in focusing it on the goal. It is able to see what is needed to get to the end goal even before your body is ready. And because of this it will work with your body until such time as it is ready.

But for some reason the word 'visualization' scares some people. Maybe it's because some of us reject the more chest-thumping motivational speakers, who advocate the technique, as a bit over the top. And yet you use visualization techniques every day of your life. It's just that you don't think of them as such.

When you look ahead to things you want, for instance your dream house, you are using this technique. You are allowing you mind to see what you want. You see the number of bedrooms you

YOUR AIM THIS WEEK

Is to visualize the details of your challenge day.

Repeat the exercise from week one, except this time picture as much as possible. 'Feel' the excitement at the start, 'smell' the air and 'hear' the noises around you. The more detail you can add in the easier it will be on the actual day of your 25 km ride.

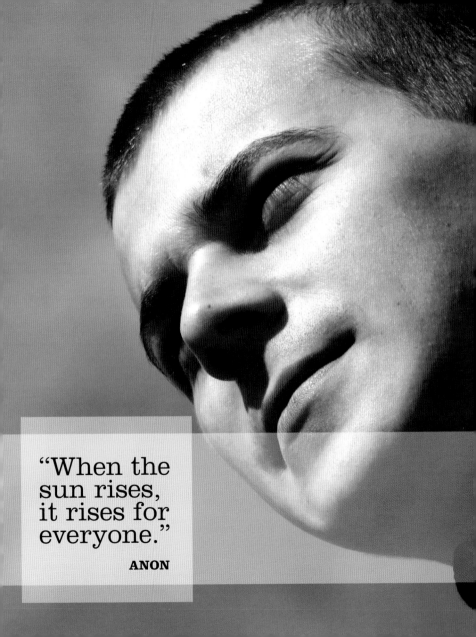

"When the sun rises, it rises for everyone."

ANON

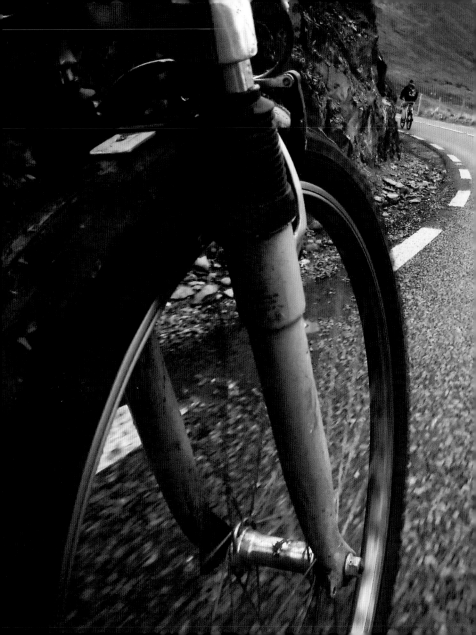

WEEK EIGHT: YOUR TRAINING PROGRAMME AND DIARY

		YOUR DAILY NOTES
MON	Rest.	
TUE	Cycle 45 mins easy to moderate. Find a 10 mins lap with at least one hill. Warm-up, stay seated uphill if you have to. Rest or spin for 2 mins. Repeat x 3.	
WED	Walk 16 mins at a moderate pace.	
THU	Rest or cross train.	
FRI	Cycle 45 mins easy-moderate. Warm-up, ride out-and-back. Easy for first 20 mins. Moderate for second 20 mins. Use last 5 mins to cool down.	
SAT	Rest.	
SUN	Cycle 55 mins easy. Ride the full distance out and back. Aim for a smooth, comfortable spin at a low-moderate effort level.	

THIS WEEK

 DO – Ensure that you eat a good snack within thirty minutes of exercise, as this is the optimum window for replenishing lost energy stores.

 CONSIDER – Checking your body position on the bike. Tuck your pelvis in to help absorb the shock. Backache is often the result of poor posture.

 DON'T – Cram-in an extra session because you missed one. Accept that your other commitments may have to come first and resume training at the next opportunity.

REWARD

A large milkshake full of goodness.

would like. You'll add in the bathrooms you'll need (en-suite for yourself maybe?). Then you'll picture the garden with the play area for the children, or the big space for the dog to run around in. Who knows, maybe there's a swimming pool somewhere in the scenario too.

If you are like most people, you'll have filled in the details too. You'll know the style of the house's architecture, the type of floors you want, even the layout and colour schemes in the rooms. You are visualizing what you want and even if you don't know it, you are setting your mind to work to achieve your dream. It might take many years but in a few years you could be living in that dream house, thanks in part to the hard work of your mind. But your mind was only able to do this because you allowed it to picture the end result (the house).

If such techniques can work on something as big as a house, it'll be a stroll in the park to use it for this 25 km cycle ride. So take a few minutes to repeat the visualization exercise, except this time fill in the details. The more you picture the details, the more comfortable you will be on the day itself. This is because you are using your 'future memory', something you have 'remembered' but which has not happened yet. Again, find somewhere quiet where you will not be disturbed, and close your eyes if this helps you to concentrate.

Sports drinks contain two important ingredients – electrolytes (they help your muscles and heart function) and carbohydrates. You can lose electrolytes through very long workouts and the carbohydrates may help provide extra energy. Try sports drinks to see if they are for you, although water will always be important for most active people. (14)

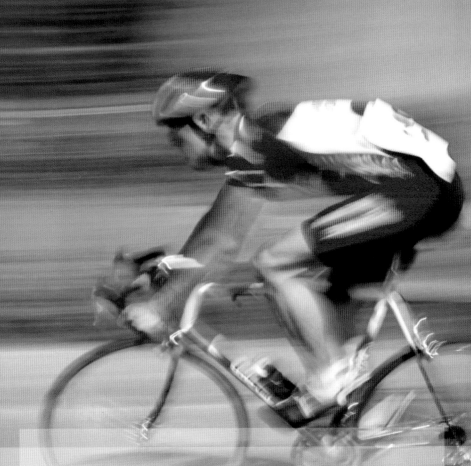

"Have the courage to follow your heart and intuition. They somehow know what you truly want to become."

STEVE JOBS

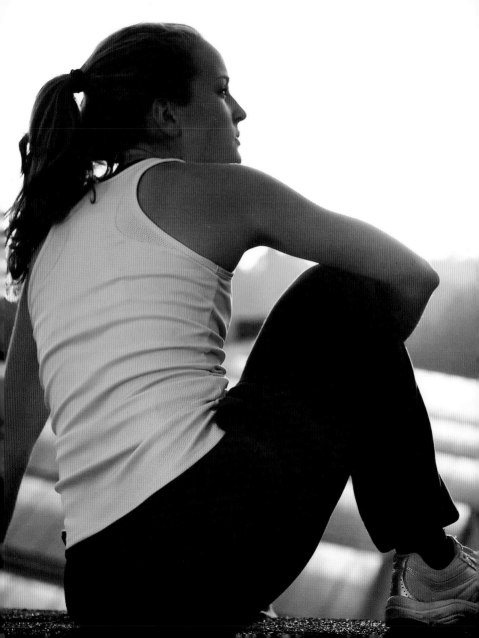

Calories in alcohol

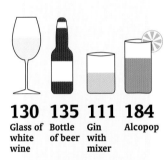

130	135	111	184
Glass of white wine	Bottle of beer	Gin with mixer	Alcopop

On a big night out it's easy to clock up the calories. The graphic shows figures for a 330 ml (11 fl oz) bottle of Stella Artois (4.8% abv), 175 ml (6 fl oz) glass of Jacob's Creek Chardonnay (13% abv), 25 ml (0.8 fl oz) of Bombay Sapphire (40% abv) and mixer, 275 ml (9 fl oz) WKD alcopop. (15)

Picture yourself getting up and preparing everything for your ride. 'See' details such as the colour of the kit you will wear. Go through the motions of 'seeing' yourself filling up your water bottle and clipping it on to your bike. Think about the type of things you might chat to your training buddy about once you have met up.

'See' yourself at the start, feeling happy and enthusiastic. 'Smell' the freshness in the air and feel the metal of your bike frame as you climb on to get going. 'Feel' comfortable as you push off and start to clock up the first few kilometres. You're soon at the halfway mark feeling strong and confident. 'Enjoy' the feeling of those pedals spinning effortlessly, as more kilometres tick by. Don't be afraid to tackle a couple of hills in your mind as you will fear them less come the day of your ride.

What are you and your training buddy chatting about as you enter the last part of your ride? 'Feel' the refreshment of the water on your lips as you take a drink. It's the last few kilometres. You've trained hard, so you have nothing to fear. Take in as many details as you can, from the sights, to the smells, to the noises. Picture yourself enjoying the last few metres, knowing nothing can stop you. Then 'feel' elated at having successfully completed the challenge and head off to 'enjoy' your reward. You've done it now, the real thing will be a doddle.

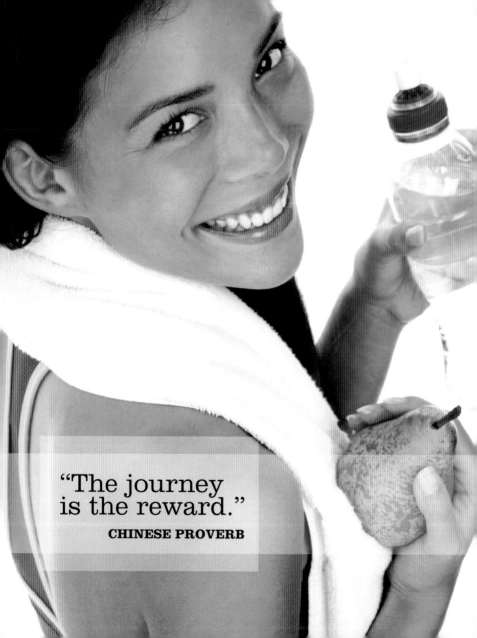

"The journey
is the reward."

CHINESE PROVERB

that's it!

Week eight completed

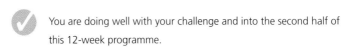 You are doing well with your challenge and into the second half of this 12-week programme.

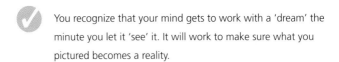 You recognize that your mind gets to work with a 'dream' the minute you let it 'see' it. It will work to make sure what you pictured becomes a reality.

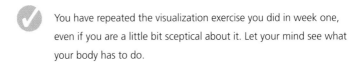 You have repeated the visualization exercise you did in week one, even if you are a little bit sceptical about it. Let your mind see what your body has to do.

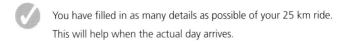 You have filled in as many details as possible of your 25 km ride. This will help when the actual day arrives.

Your notes at the
end of the week

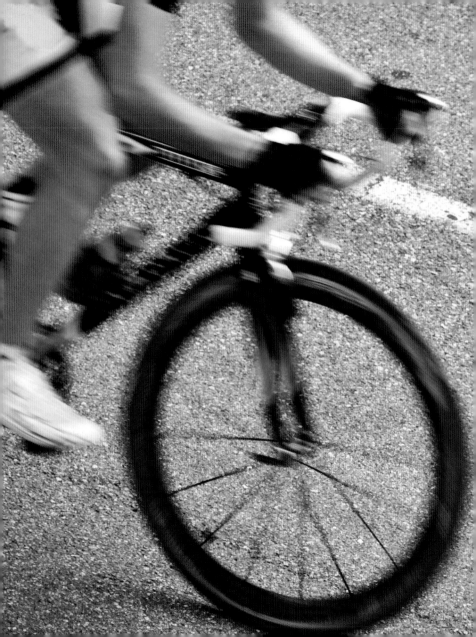

week nine

The end goal is in sight

It's time to push on towards the finish...

At the start of this programme everything was about motivation and simply climbing on to the bike again. You probably had enough to contend with just getting into the groove of changing gears without looking down. But slowly these basics will have returned to you and your cycling will have soon become a way of getting fit.

Now you are back into the groove (you don't still look down when you change gears do you?), you can afford to spend a bit of time looking at your technique. There's no need to become a cycling guru overnight, but a few minutes could save you valuable effort and improve your speeds.

First up, nobody likes hills, so you are not alone there. One minute you are cruising along at one with the world, happily enjoying yourself, then you turn the corner to see a long climb ahead of you. However, it's virtually impossible to cycle without going up sometimes, so hills are something you have to deal with. Who knows, you may even approach them as a

YOUR AIM THIS WEEK

Is to look closer at your technique and mental approach, to see how this can help your cycling.

Just looking at some basic things, with regards to uphills, downhills and your pedal stroke, could reduce your effort levels but still lead to an increase in your cycling speeds.

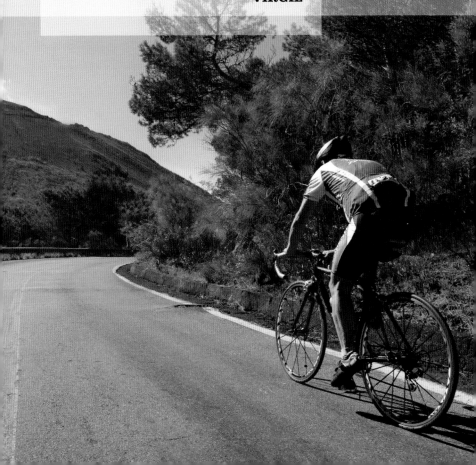

"They succeed
because they think
they can."

VIRGIL

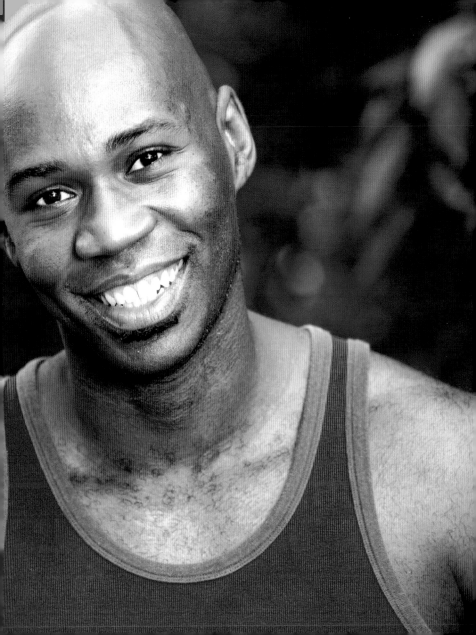

WEEK NINE: YOUR TRAINING PROGRAMME AND DIARY

		YOUR DAILY NOTES
MON	Rest.	
TUE	Cycle 35 mins easy-moderate. Warm-up, ride for 8 mins. Focus on a smooth, comfortable stroke. Rest or spin for 2 mins. Repeat x 3.	
WED	Walk for 10 mins at a moderate pace.	
THU	Rest or cross train.	
FRI	Cycle 35 mins easy-moderate. Warm-up, ride for 6 mins at a comfortable pace. Increase effort level for last 30 secs. Rest or spin for 2 mins. Repeat x 4.	
SAT	Rest.	
SUN	Cycle 45 mins easy.	

THIS WEEK

 DO – Maintain a healthy ratio in your diet: carbohydrates – 50%, protein – 30%, fats – 20%.

 CONSIDER – Watching less TV and read a book instead.

 DON'T – Fill up on junk food prior to exercise. What you eat has a huge bearing on your performance out on the road.

REWARD

Have a cheat day. Eat and drink whatever you want.

challenge one day? As you approach a hill don't forget the basics of getting your bike into the correct gear. You should do this while you are on the flat and not when you hit the hill. If you time it too late you'll find yourself battling up the slope in too high a gear and forced to a virtual standstill. Even professional cyclists can get this wrong sometimes, so practise your timing so you'll always head into the hills with momentum.

More than ever this is the time to concentrate on maintaining a smooth pedal stroke and avoid jerking through the 'dead spots' we mentioned earlier. When cycling uphill try to maintain an even level of effort and just accept it's natural that you will slow down. Whatever you do, don't 'attack' the slope. This is a subconscious effort to 'beat the hill' or at least 'get it over with as quickly as possible'. While this is a perfectly natural tendency, it's not a good one. Hills are all about a steady effort.

Don't be tempted to stop, or slow down in relief at 'having made it', when you do get to the top. Keep going at the same effort level and you will quickly regain your breath. Finally, if you do find yourself pushing your bike up part of the hill, or all of it, even at this stage in the programme, then that's fine, as you will continue to improve over the coming weeks.

Avoid the temptation to lean forward as the power comes from you being centred and driving down

4 or 9

Sugars and starches (carbohydrates) found in foods such as pasta, bread, cereal, fruit and vegetables have four calories per gram (0.14 oz) while fat is more than double at nine calories per gram (0.32 oz). Worth knowing when you're trying to get fit and healthy don't you reckon? (16)

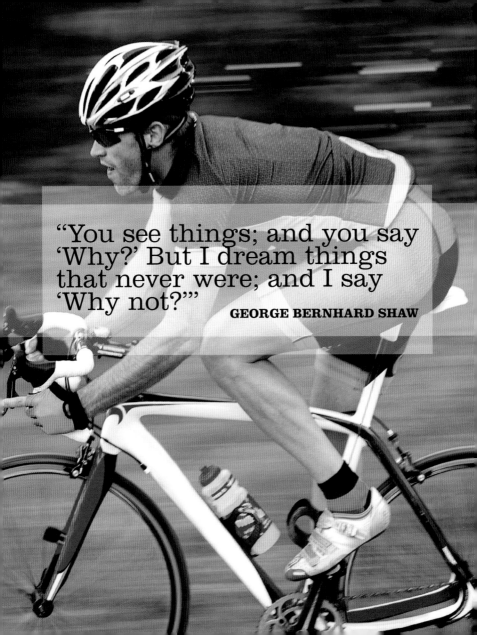

"You see things; and you say
'Why?' But I dream things
that never were; and I say
'Why not?'"   GEORGE BERNHARD SHAW

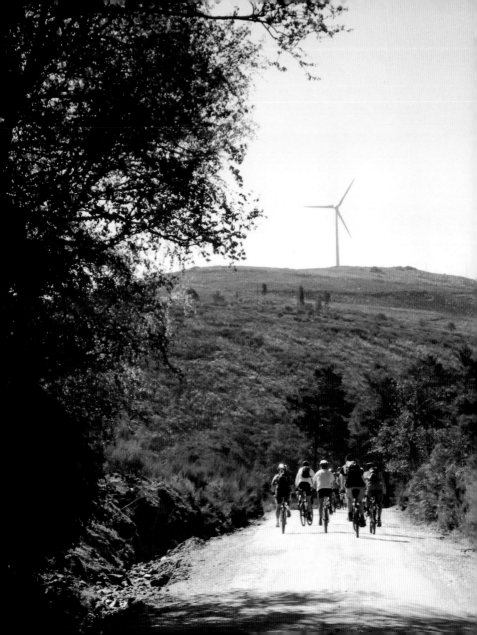

through the bike. Also avoid standing up out of the saddle, as this forces up your heart rate. Although this may be necessary on particularly steep sections, make sure you limit these tiring bursts.

Then there are the downhill sections. It's always lovely to see a nice downhill stretch ahead. When you are tired this gives you a welcome break and it's also a good way to get a few easy metres out the way. Bear in mind that your body will naturally get pitched forward when you are going downhill, so concentrate on keeping centred over your bike for both balance and control.

The main thing when going downhill is to feel safe and, especially when cornering. By all means lower your body down into a streamlined positioned if it is more comfortable, but make sure you build your confidence slowly with your speed. Remember the faster you are going, the less time you have to react, and the less control you will have over your bike. Don't be afraid to ease up if you feel uncomfortable with your speed at any time.

Keep your hands close to the brakes but avoid applying them too sharply, unless you are really fond of laying on Tarmac. Potholes and loose stones can also cause accidents so always keep your eyes open for obstacles such as these, and in a race, of course, for other cyclists.

A balanced diet

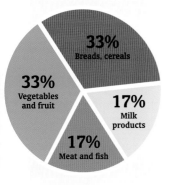

33%
Breads, cereals

33%
Vegetables and fruit

17%
Milk products

17%
Meat and fish

Try to maintain a balanced diet of the 'basic four food groups' in the proportions shown in the chart above and to eat from all of them every day. Also limit the amount of fats you include in your diet. (17)

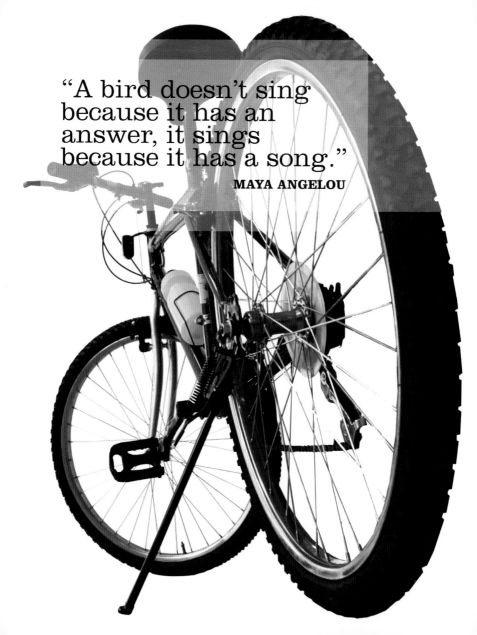

"A bird doesn't sing because it has an answer, it sings because it has a song."

MAYA ANGELOU

that's it!

Week nine completed

 You know it is worth spending a few minutes thinking about your technique during your training.

 You know it is particularly important to get into the correct gear as you approach the hill and not once you are on it. Time it wrong and you'll find yourself at a standstill.

 You know it is important to maintain an even level of effort when cycling uphill and accept you will slow down. Don't try 'to beat' the hills.

 You will naturally generate more speed as you cycle downhill, but build your confidence slowly with your downhill speeds.

Your notes at the
end of the week

Keep focused on your goal

Beware the spectre of over-confidence. It can kill all your hard work…

Who would have thought a few weeks ago, as you took those first, tentative pedal strokes, that we would be warning you against over-confidence. But at this stage, as the finish becomes so tantalizingly close, over-confidence can be a real danger.

When you have just dragged yourself from the armchair after a long absence from exercise, improvement can be rapid. It feels good, both physically and mentally, and you can rightly feel proud of how much you have achieved so quickly. But with this comes a feeling that you can conquer anything. Enjoy the feeling but don't lose sight of reality. Nine weeks of training does not make you ready for the Tour de France.

Over-confidence is like a nasty little pest sitting on your shoulder, urging you on to do more. "Don't take notice of your book. You are king of the road. Cycle more, cycle harder. Squeeze in another session. You are the king of the road."

YOUR AIM THIS WEEK

Is to be careful of becoming over-confident and doing extra training.

By all means enjoy what you have achieved, but remember you are aiming for a 25 km ride in two weeks. There is no point over doing it now and draining yourself for the main event.

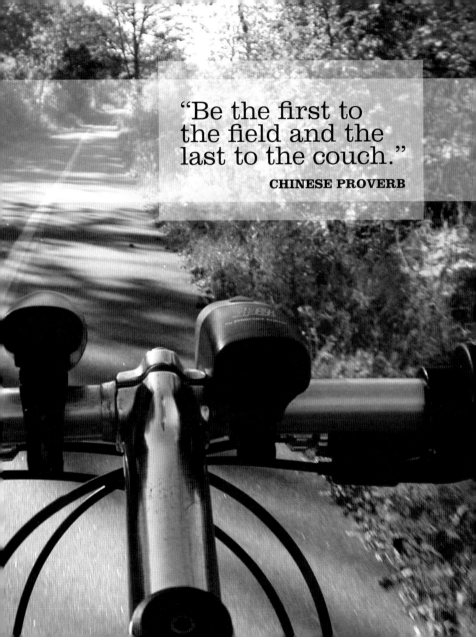

"Be the first to the field and the last to the couch."

CHINESE PROVERB

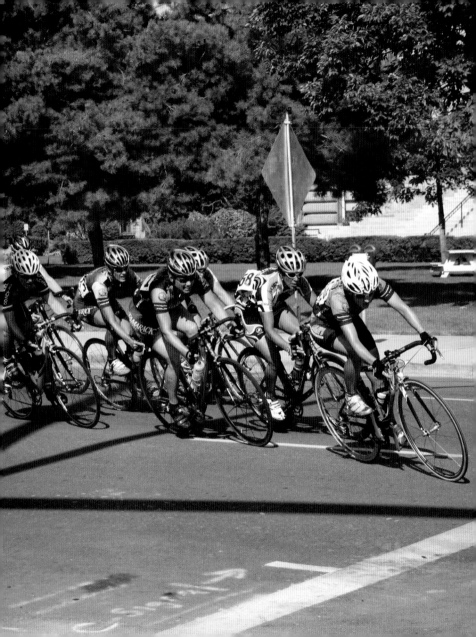

		YOUR DAILY NOTES
MON	Rest. This is your final week of high volume, so take it easy.	
TUE	Cycle 50 mins easy-moderate. Warm-up, find a 12 mins lap with at least one hill. Stay seated uphill if you have to. Rest or spin for 2 mins. Repeat x 3.	
WED	Walk 16 mins at a moderate pace.	
THU	Rest or cross train.	
FRI	Cycle 50 mins easy-moderate. Warm-up for 5 mins, ride easy for first 20 mins, moderate for second 20 mins. Use last 5 mins to cool down.	
SAT	Rest.	
SUN	Cycle 60 mins easy.	

THIS WEEK

 DO – Tell friends and family about your progress. You'll be surprised at how inspired people are when you share your goals.

 CONSIDER – Using puncture-resistant tyres, as these can save you valuable time and heartache when you're out training.

 DON'T – Lose sight of your target – to cycle 25 km without stopping.

REWARD

Treat yourself to a spa and sauna.

Flip that little pest off your shoulder and squish him (he's not real, so no harm done). You have followed the programme carefully up until now (we hope), so stick to it to the end. If you let the over-confidence pest get the better of you it will go like this…

You head out on your bike, as usual, for one of your training sessions (let's say Tuesday, where you will be repeating a 12-minute lap, including a hill, repeated three times). The pace should be easy to moderate, so after your stretch and warm-up you complete the first lap comfortably. During your rest period (two minutes), you realize you are feeling stronger than usual. "Maybe it was that nice sleep I had last night," you think to yourself.

You wonder if you could do the same lap a bit quicker, maybe knock 30 seconds off it? So you do. In the next two-minute break you feel as if someone has dropped the Superman cloak over you. "That sleep really was good," you conclude, as you head off, this time determined to see just how fast you can complete the same lap.

You push it from the start, keep pushing even when you legs feel heavy and drained, but you finish quickly and you beam a big smile at the end. And why not? You have proved how much your hard work over the last few weeks is paying off. But the trouble is, your goal is not to complete a lap in record time in

17-19

Researchers in Australia and New Zealand found that people who drove after being awake for 17-19 hours performed worse than those who had a blood-alcohol level of 0.5 per cent – the legal limit for drivers in Australia and many European countries. It's not difficult to see that sleep is important for anyone who wants to focus on his/her health and fitness. (18)

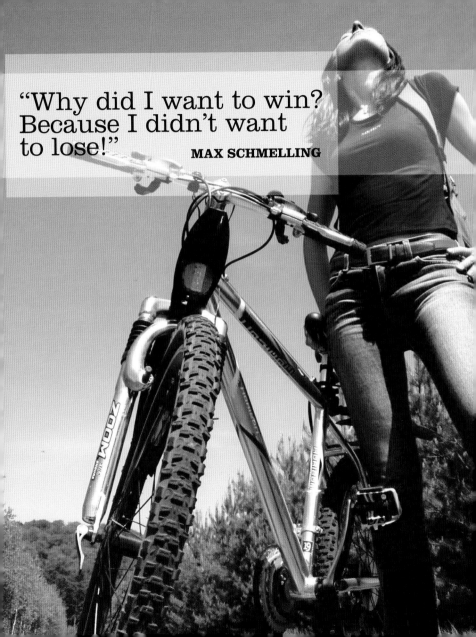

"Why did I want to win? Because I didn't want to lose!"

MAX SCHMELLING

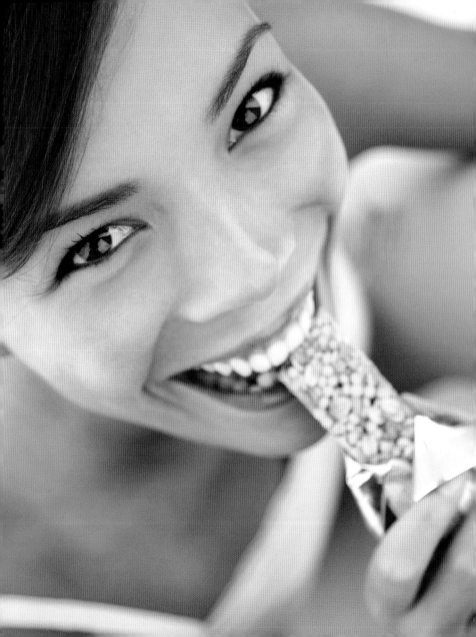

The human body

60%
Water

40%
Other

Around 55-60 per cent of your body is made up of water. Your brain is 70 per cent water, blood 83 per cent water and lungs nearly 90 per cent. Make sure you keep yourself topped up by drinking plenty of water throughout the day. (19)

Week 10. Your goal is to complete a 25 km cycle ride in Week 12.

All you have actually achieved is to drain your body of the energy it needs to complete your real goal. Training is all about building up gradually to peak at the right time, but in this scenario all you have done is knocked yourself backwards. If you do something like this there is a real chance you may fail to finish the challenge altogether. Be very careful about over-confidence, no matter how good you feel, and stick to the training as set out in the programme.

Other things to be wary of at this stage are injury and illness. The good news is that moderate exercise makes it less likely for you to pick up a bug. However, continue to follow all the normal rules you do to avoid a cold, such as keeping warm (especially after a workout), washing your hands regularly, and eating and sleeping well. Time is tight now, so you really do not need to be laid up in bed.

Injuries can be kept at bay by keeping your training steady (none of those over-confidence bursts now) and by maintaining your stretching regime. Keep stretching before and after every workout, and try to do a bit extra on your rest days. If, despite your efforts, you do fall ill or pick up an injury, rest until you are fully recovered. If necessary consult a doctor or physio. Do not train when sick or injured.

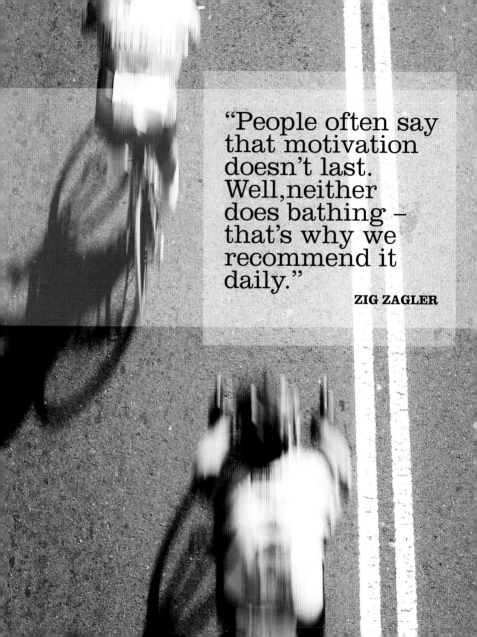

"People often say that motivation doesn't last. Well, neither does bathing – that's why we recommend it daily."

ZIG ZAGLER

that's it!

Week ten completed

 You are feeling strong and fit after so much hard work. Enjoy it, but keep focused as there is still some work to do.

 You know that no matter how good you feel you should be wary of over-confidence. This can lead to you pushing yourself too hard in a training session, or doing an extra session. Avoid this as it could drain you for your main goal – the 25 km ride.

 You will do everything you can to avoid sickness or injury so your plans are not derailed. Eat well, sleep well, and remember to keep stretching out your muscles.

 You know that if you do get sick or injured, however, you should rest until you have recovered. Consult a doctor or physio if necessary but do not keep training.

Your notes at the end of the week

week eleven

Now ease up

With your challenge day so close you can start winding down…

The good thing about most exercise programmes (and this one is no different), is that as you get close to your goal you can start to ease up. This is because the hard work has already been done, the kilometres are in your legs, and now you need to conserve energy for the end goal – your 25 km ride.

So this week the time you spend exercising will decrease. Your two rides in the week (Tuesday and Friday) are down from 50 minutes to 40 minutes each, while your longer distance ride (Sunday) drops 10 minutes from last week to a total of 50 minutes. Your easy, loosener walk, is down a few minutes as well, and while you can still cross train on Thursday if you want to, remember to keep all workouts at a relaxed tempo.

Nerves can creep in at this stage. They'll be triggered by the things we've already discussed: thoughts that you've not done enough, or you've done too much, and so on. But your nerves are just a natural

YOUR AIM THIS WEEK

Is to avoid taking on new projects from your 'to do' list.

When a goal or target approaches it is common for people to do something to distract themselves. This is down to nerves, but it should be avoided. Concentrate on the task at hand so you mind and body is ready.

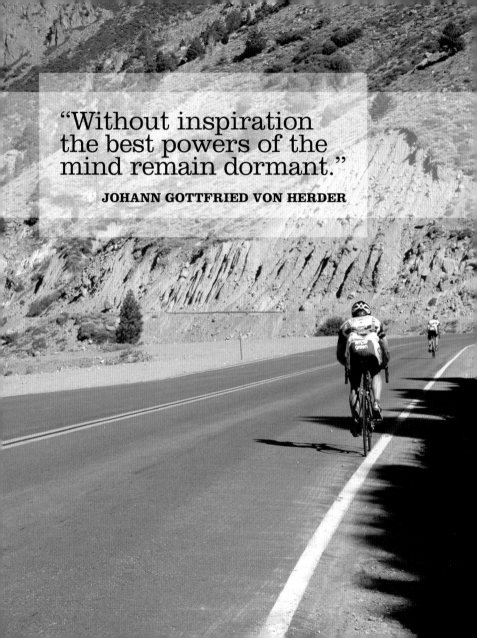

"Without inspiration the best powers of the mind remain dormant."

JOHANN GOTTFRIED VON HERDER

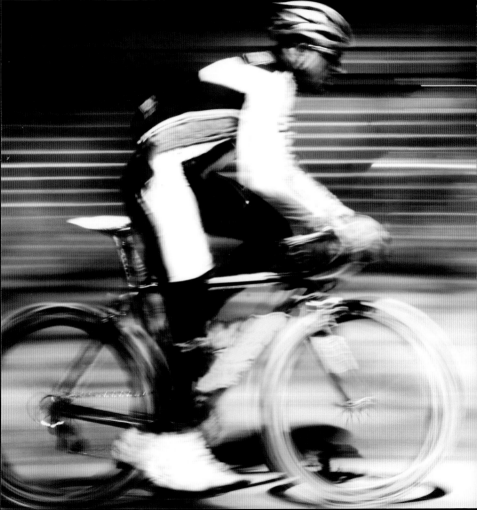

WEEK ELEVEN: YOUR TRAINING PROGRAMME AND DIARY

		YOUR DAILY NOTES
MON	Rest. Exercise volume begins to decrease from now until your goal.	
TUE	Cycle 40 mins easy-moderate. Find a hilly course. Warm-up, try to keep your heart rate down on the flats. Conserve energy.	
WED	Walk for 12 mins at a moderate pace.	
THU	Rest or cross train.	
FRI	Cycle 40 mins easy-moderate. Warm-up, ride for 4 mins easy then 1 min moderate. Repeat x 6.	
SAT	Rest.	
SUN	Cycle 50 mins easy.	

THIS WEEK

 DO – Elevate your legs when you're at home, to rest your leg muscles and aid circulation.

 CONSIDER – Adding swimming to your cross training (if you haven't already) as the water is great for fitness recovery.

 DON'T – Forget the importance of warming-up and cooling down before and after exercise.

REWARD

Buy a new
set of tyres
for your bike.

part of approaching any target or goal. The closer a target gets, the more real it gets, and that's when your nerves creep in. Keep reminding yourself you have followed a programme that has been carefully worked out and you have nothing to worry about.

Your life is probably busy with work and family commitments, so as much as possible, keep your mind focused on the 25 km target ride. Limit your commitments if you can. While you're not going to be able to live, breathe and sleep your ride like a professional cyclist, concentrate on the things you can control and try not to worry about the things you can't.

36°C

You will still have reports that need filing at work, the children will still need picking up from school, and mum will still want her regular chats on the phone. These are things you can't control, so deal with them as you have always dealt with them. But there are some things you can control.

Be particularly careful when exercising in hot weather. Once the temperature rises to 36°C (97°F) it is recommended you cancel your session or postpone it to a cooler part of the day as the heat will put a lot of stress on your body. [20]

The main thing is to avoid taking on a new project at this stage. We all have a long list of things we want to do. You know the type of things: learn a foreign language, play an instrument like a professional, or sign up for a pottery course at your local college. While all of these are laudable (and we are sure you'll do them all one day), let the list stay quiet for a bit longer. After all, if you haven't started

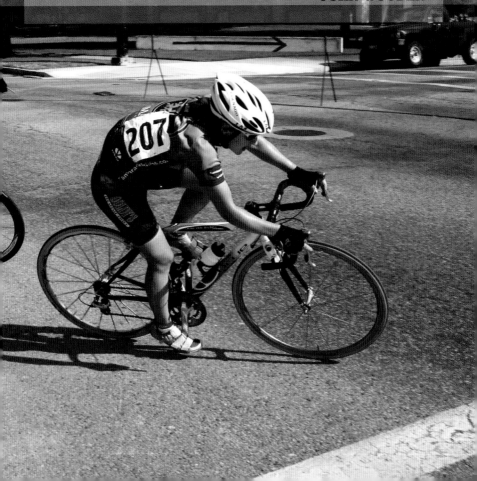

"Sports do not build character.
They reveal it."

JOHN WOODEN

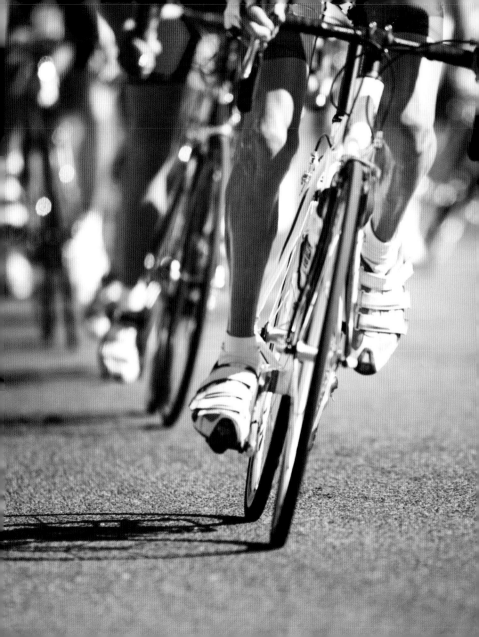

A balanced meal

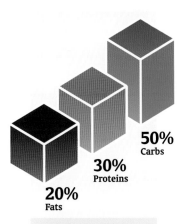

50%
Carbs

30%
Proteins

20%
Fats

Try to balance all food elements with every meal you eat in line with the figures shown in the chart above.

Carbohydrates include rice, bread, fruits and vegetables, proteins come from meat, fish, milk products and eggs, while nuts, avocados, green olives, fish oil and olive oil are a good source of fats. (21)

on those Spanish-as-a-foreign-language tapes for two years is it really that important you get stuck into them right now?

The reason you might be tempted to get stuck into your list at this stage is to distract yourself from your nerves. It's okay, this is a perfectly normal reaction. But avoid touching the list (at least until after you have finished that 25 km ride). Right now you need to keep what you are doing to the minimum and focus on your big ride.

With only a few days to go you should also be concentrating on getting good sleep every night, keeping hydrated, eating well in the day, and easing up on the alcohol.

Remember the best sleep is regular sleep where you go to bed at the same time and get up at the same time every day. Even if you haven't done this until now, try to do it for the next few days leading up to your 25 km ride. Keep drinking water during the day (you are hopefully already into this habit). If the water cooler at work is a fair walk up the corridor then fill up a bottle and leave it on your desk for easy access. And while we are not suggesting you become a monk on the alcohol front (a glass of wine after work won't hurt you), this is probably not the time to be embarking on a series of big nights with your wildest friend. There will be plenty of time to celebrate.

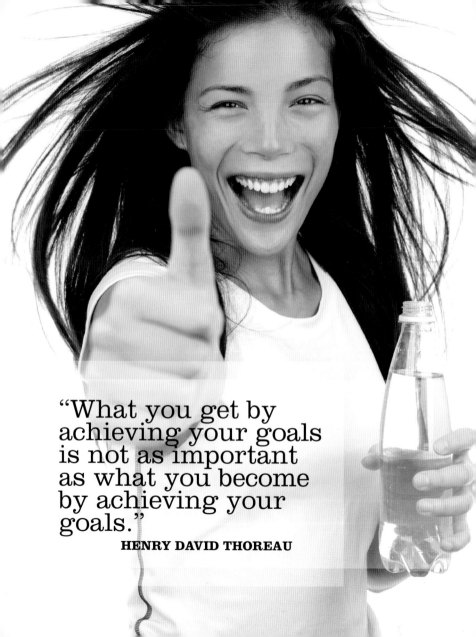

"What you get by achieving your goals is not as important as what you become by achieving your goals."

HENRY DAVID THOREAU

that's it!

Week eleven completed

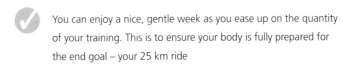 You can enjoy a nice, gentle week as you ease up on the quantity of your training. This is to ensure your body is fully prepared for the end goal – your 25 km ride

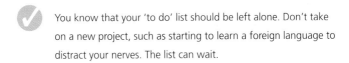 You know that your 'to do' list should be left alone. Don't take on a new project, such as starting to learn a foreign language to distract your nerves. The list can wait.

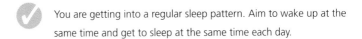 You are getting into a regular sleep pattern. Aim to wake up at the same time and get to sleep at the same time each day.

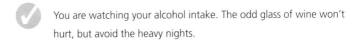 You are watching your alcohol intake. The odd glass of wine won't hurt, but avoid the heavy nights.

Your notes at the end of the week

week twelve

Get ready to ride

**After many weeks of hard training you are
ready for your challenge…**

So the moment has arrived. This is the week of
your challenge. Enjoy the feeling of anticipation as
the big ride approaches. Remind yourself that you
are physically and mentally ready because you have
followed the programme. All that remains is to
complete your 25 km ride.

There are only a couple of sessions this week and
these are intended to keep you loose for the big ride.
Keep the tempo nice and easy on Tuesday (your last
ride before the challenge). Apart from this there is
only a walk (Wednesday), plus an optional cross-
training session (Thursday) planned for this week.
Otherwise, rest up so you are fresh. Lots of stretching,
as always, is recommended.

Get everything you will need ready ahead of the day
itself so there are no last-minute panics. You don't
need to be searching for your water bottle on the
morning of your ride. Go through the checklist below
to make sure you are well prepared.

YOUR AIM THIS WEEK

Is to successfully complete
your challenge of a 25 km
ride. This is what you have
worked for.

Enjoy this last week in the
lead up to the big ride,
content in the knowledge
that if you have followed
the programme then you
are ready.

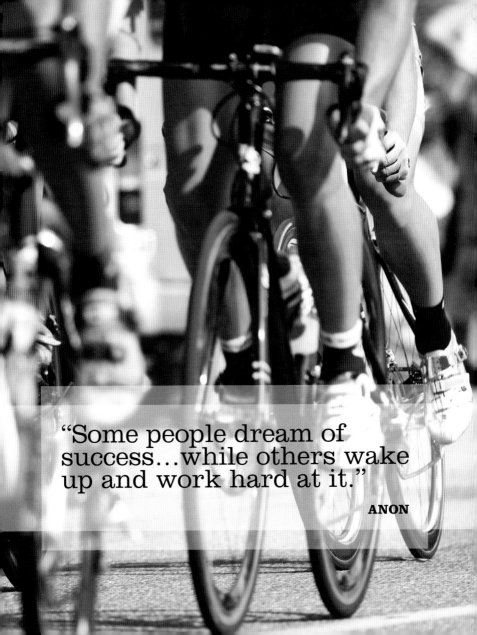

"Some people dream of success…while others wake up and work hard at it."

ANON

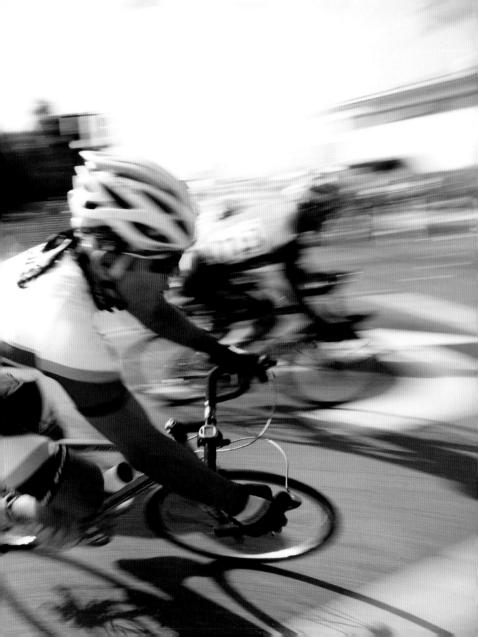

WEEK TWELVE: YOUR TRAINING PROGRAMME AND DIARY

YOUR DAILY NOTES

MON	Rest.
TUE	Cycle 30 mins easy-moderate. Warm-up, ride easy first 15 mins, moderate second 15 mins. Use last 5 mins to cool down.
WED	Walk 10 mins at a moderate pace.
THU	Rest or easy cross train (eg. a gentle swim).
FRI	Rest.
SAT	Your 25 km race or rest. Choose the day which suits you best.
SUN	Your 25 km race or rest. Choose the day which suits you best.

THIS WEEK

DO – Enjoy this last week of your training.

CONSIDER – Buying a bike rack, so you can drive out to scenic cycling routes, away from heavy traffic.

DON'T – Forget your drinks bottle to mount on your bike.

REWARD

Congratulate yourself on successfully completing your goal!

Checklist

- ☐ Cycling shoes
- ☐ Socks
- ☐ Padded shorts
- ☐ Cycling top
- ☐ Wind jacket
- ☐ Cap or peak
- ☐ Sunglasses
- ☐ Sun cream
- ☐ Water bottle or sports drink
- ☐ Energy bar
- ☐ Race number, safety pins
- ☐ Map and transport details for getting to the start
- ☐ Towel and wet wipes

It's not unusual to struggle to sleep the night before a big event, so try to get as much quality sleep as you can in the nights leading up to it. On the night before the ride have a good dinner, but nothing too heavy, and avoid caffeine and alcohol as these will disturb your sleep.

Have breakfast and a glass of water at least an hour before the planned start of your ride. Stick to food you are used to (both the night before and in the morning) so as not to upset your stomach. You can experiment with new dishes later! Run through the details of your race one more time in your mind, remembering to picture success all the way.

If you did manage to find an organized race for your challenge everything may be a little daunting, especially if you have never been in a race before. Make sure you arrive in plenty of time so you can get you bearings, and listen to any briefings that may

6-10

If you need a performance boost in the day then a short sleep – or a power nap if you want to sound smart – of just six to 10 minutes could do the trick. If this sounds like something for you then keep the nap short and sharp so you avoid waking up feeling groggy. (22)

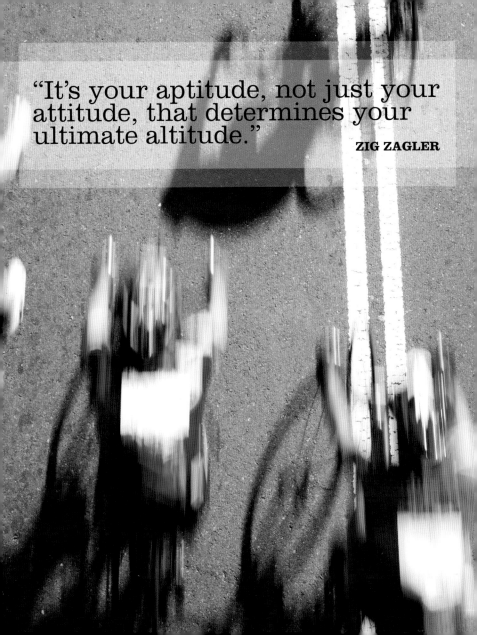

"It's your aptitude, not just your attitude, that determines your ultimate altitude."

ZIG ZAGLER

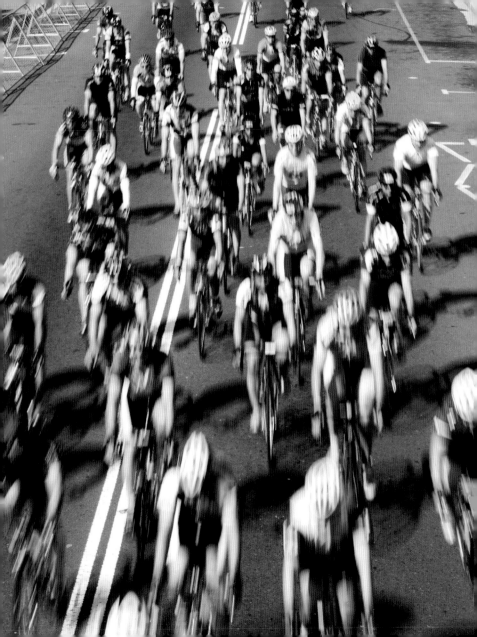

be issued by race officials. You will feel a sense of excitement in the air so soak up the atmosphere and enjoy yourself. Don't, however, get carried away and go riding off at a pace that is too quick.

It is easy to get caught up in the excitement but keep focused on your own race and do not worry about other cyclists around you. Take no notice if it seems other riders are passing you because you are riding your own race. The slower starters are often strong at the end, anyway, so there is a good chance you will be passing many of these cyclists later on.

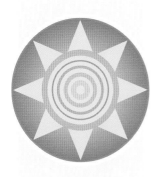

In the bigger races with lots of cyclists it is likely the course will get congested. Keep an eye open for riders ahead of you slowing down or stopping suddenly. Move gradually and carefully to the edge of the road if you need to stop.

Have you ever noticed how refreshed and good you feel after exercising once the huffing and puffing has stopped?

Numerous studies have found there is a direct link between exercising and feeling happy and satisfied with your life. Getting a smile on your face – can there be a better reason for you to exercise? (23)

If you set up your own 'race' then still treat it as a special event – after all, you have worked hard for this – and make sure you have enough water for the ride. If you have a training buddy for your challenge then chat about your ride as this will help calm your nerves. Talk through the route and remind each other of the reward you have set up when you successfully complete the ride.

You are ready, so go out with a smile on your face and enjoy your ride!

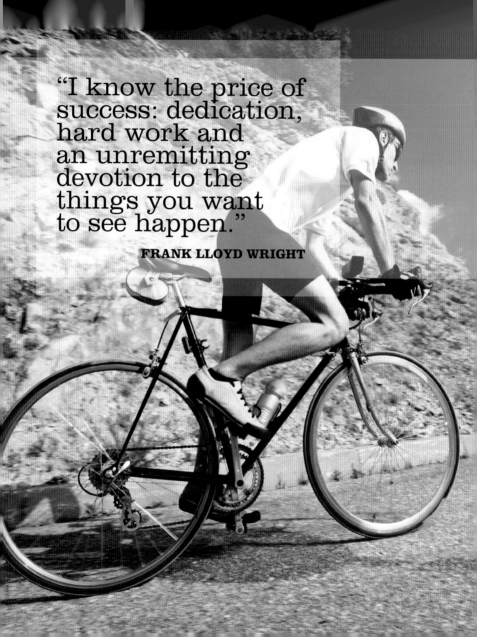

"I know the price of success: dedication, hard work and an unremitting devotion to the things you want to see happen."

FRANK LLOYD WRIGHT

that's it!

Week twelve completed

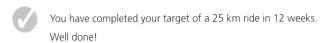

You have completed your target of a 25 km ride in 12 weeks. Well done!

You can congratulate yourself on what you have achieved in a relatively short time.

Your hard work has made you fitter and healthier. Enjoy the feeling and keep working hard. It's easier to stay fit than it is to get fit in the first place.

You need to go and enjoy your reward. Whatever it is you have chosen, remind yourself that you deserve it.

Your notes at the
end of the week

what now?

You can now look ahead

Your 25 km ride is successfully behind you.
Now, what…

Hands up if you want to pack all this exercise stuff in right now, slump back into your comfortable armchair and order a double-cheese pizza with garlic bread on the side. Mmm, we must admit, the pizza sounds good, but it really would be a waste to stop now wouldn't it?

The good news is that you have done all the hard work already. The difficult bit, when getting fit, is simply starting, then working through the first few sessions. These can be tough (as you may remember) because you body will be creaking and groaning after so long away from exercising. But once you've shaken that rustiness out of your muscles your body starts to play ball. This is where you are now

So pack it in if you want. After all, you have proved to yourself, and all the other doubters, that you can do it. But it might be a better idea, now you've done all the groundwork, to keep at it, or even push on from here to see just how fit you can get.

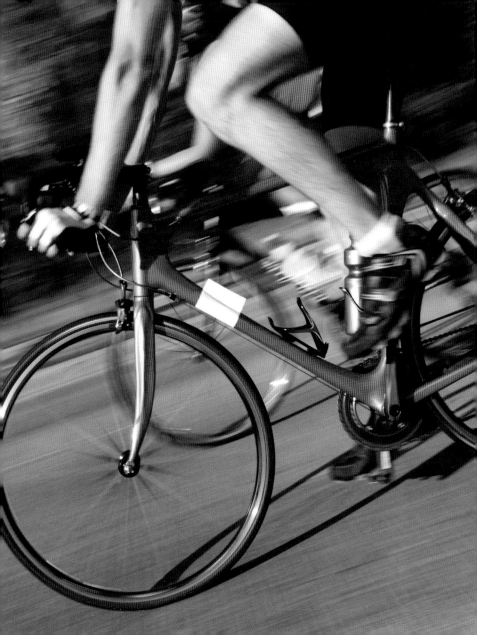

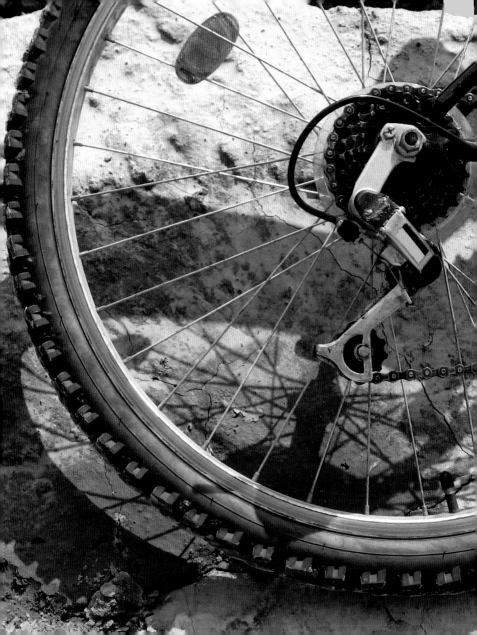

It's easy enough to continue to enjoy the benefits of your new-found fitness – sleeping better, waking up more refreshed, and not feeling sluggish during the day – by just maintaining your current level of training. At least you know you can fit in this amount of training each week.

It helps if you set yourself a challenge, as this gives you something to aim for (in the same way as the programme in this book has guided you towards your 25 km ride). Find a similar challenge to the one you have just completed (or maybe a longer distance this time) if that's what you need to inspire you. Maybe you could look at joining a local cycling club if you are really getting into your riding. Training with other people with similar aims will keep you energized.

But don't be afraid to mix it up and start a new activity. Remember, there's no rule that says you have to only cycle. Spend some time swimming, running, or dancing – whatever it is that keeps you motivated and keeps you fit.

If you do feel yourself losing motivation in the future then tune your mind into the success you have enjoyed in this programme. Read back over your notes to remind yourself of how quickly you improved. In particular, think of the benefits you are enjoying from being fit and healthy. But there's a good chance you are feeling on top of the world right now and are starting to aim for bigger things (100-kilometre races and the like). You have every right to, but be warned not to take on more than you can handle in terms of time. It wasn't that long ago that the pressures of time (probably) stopped you from exercising altogether. There is no point in taking on a challenge that requires you to train for three hours a day, six days a week if you simply don't have the time to do it.

In the euphoria of finishing a challenge it's common to set new goals (a good thing) but keep them realistic. Make sure the new targets you set are achievable or you could fall behind in your schedule. This can lead to demotivation and the possibility of giving up altogether (a bad thing). It is better to keep doing a few quality training sessions than attempt to do too much and fail.

Whatever you decide to do next you can take comfort in the fact that you have set yourself a target and, after some hard work, you have successfully completed it. This is something you can carry forward, not only in terms of fitness, but also in other areas of your life. Keep drawing on the success of the last 12 weeks.

So, congratulations at having successfully completed your 25 km cycle challenge and good luck with your next challenge, whatever it may be.

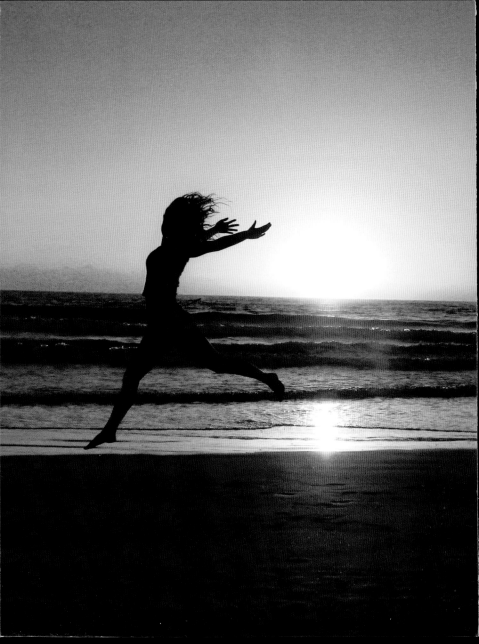

First published in 2013 by
New Holland Publishers (UK) Ltd
London • Cape Town • Sydney • Auckland
www.newhollandpublishers.com

A catalogue record for this book is available from the British Library.

ISBN 978 1 78009 2348

This book has been produced for New Holland Publishers by
Chase My Snail Ltd
London • Cape Town
www.chasemysnail.com

Designer: Darren Exell
Photo Editor: Anthony Ernest
Proof readers: David Chapman, Tony Headley
Consultant sports psychologist: Russell Murphy
Production: Marion Storz

2 4 6 8 10 9 7 5 3 1

Printed and bound in China by Toppan Leefung Printing Ltd.